Neo-shamanism and Mental Health

Karel James Bouse

Neo-shamanism and Mental Health

palgrave
macmillan

Karel James Bouse
Institute of Esoteric Psychology
Loudon, TN, USA

ISBN 978-3-030-31910-6 ISBN 978-3-030-31911-3 (eBook)
https://doi.org/10.1007/978-3-030-31911-3

This Palgrave Pivot imprint is published by the registered company Springer Nature Switzerland AG
The registered company address is: Gewerbestrasse 11, 6330 Cham, Switzerland

This book is dedicated in thanks to Drs. Stanley Krippner, Ruth Richards, and Jacquie Lewis.

Introduction

Journeys bring power and love back into you. —Rumi

This book is about the ancient technology of shamanism and its potential application in contemporary life as a means of enhancing wellbeing by integrating mind, body and spirit, and strengthening one's connection to nature, the sacred and the self. It examines traditional shamanism and Neo-shamanism in order to differentiate the two practices which are simultaneously similar and different. It details a research study undertaken in 2017 which examined the practices, beliefs and lifeworlds of some contemporary Neo-shamanic practitioners in order to serve as a basis for understanding how Neo-shamanism functions in contemporary Western culture. The book allows these practitioners to describe their lifeworlds through their own recorded journeys and responses to deeply personal interview questions. It explores the potential value that the ancient technology of the shamanic journey might have as part of a controlled phenomenological qualitative research protocol for consciousness studies, and how it might benefit self-exploration as part of a supervised multi-modal wellness curriculum or therapy. Further, there is a discussion about the possible pitfalls present in contemporary Neo-shamanic practice, including the effects of cultural dissonance and spiritual bypassing. Finally the book engages in exploring the way in which Neo-shamanic practices might act as a viable adjunct to standard clinical therapeutic practice.

Neo-shamanism and Mental Health is an examination and discussion of contemporary Neo-shamanic practice and the mental health benefits that might be derived from its application to the mental health field. It is based on peer-reviewed literature, the results of a 2017 research project investigating the lifeworlds of six American Neo-shamanic practitioners, and my own observations as a student, teacher, and practitioner of Neo-shamanism for nearly three decades. Chapter 1 explores and discusses the similarities and differences between traditional and/or indigenous shamanism and contemporary Western Neo-shamanism. Chapter 2 is an overview of the method and results of the 2017 research project and protocol, including reproduction of the research instruments. Chapter 3 focuses on the lifeworlds of the 2017 participants, each of which offers an intimate and detailed glimpse into rich alternative worldviews and individual expanded consciousness. Chapter 4 outlines the multi-modal teaching template for shamanic journey-based self-discovery that I have used in classes and workshops with excellent results, and which has the potential to be equally beneficial as part of a therapeutic setting when deemed appropriate. Chapter 5 delves into the psychological pitfalls of cultural dissonance, dysfunctional identity, and spiritual bypassing that might befall ill-trained, undisciplined, and unsupervised Neo-shamanic practitioners, especially those lacking the requisite self-knowledge and awareness. Chapter 6 discusses how the shamanic journey technology could be applied as a tool to gather phenomenological data as an aid to consciousness studies as part of a controlled and replicable laboratory research protocol. Chapter 7 is an overview of the conclusions derived from the preceding chapters, as well as presenting possible avenues of further inquiry. It also examines the potential benefits of using Neo-shamanic practice as an adjunct to standard therapeutic practices. Anomalous findings discovered through such research might hold the potential to instigate a paradigm shift away from our sensory-cognitive based concept of reality and toward expanded models of consciousness and accepted reality constructs.

Glossary of Terms

There are some specific terms used repeatedly throughout this book. Below is a Glossary of the most frequently used terms to facilitate clear communication and understanding of the material.

Altered State of Consciousness (ASC): The term "altered state of consciousness" refers to any psychological state different from normal waking consciousness. Although dreaming is an altered state of consciousness, the ASCs under discussion here are those in which the individual retains liminal awareness and the ability to perceive phenomena usually imperceptible while in the normal waking state (Rock & Krippner, 2007; VandenBos, 2015).

Anomalous Experience: Refers to any experience or set of experiences that fall outside of the parameters and explanations of rational, sensory-based material cognition and societal reality constructs. These include out-of-body experiences, mystical experiences, shamanic journeys, and interactions with anomalous phenomena (VandenBos, 2015).

Dasein: *Dasein* is the term used by Martin Heidegger to describe a way of being manifested as human that enables us to inquire into the mysteries of being, and the manner in which they might perceive and exist in the world (VandenBos, 2015). *Dasein* also incorporates the process of one's "becoming" (p. 282).

Lifeworld: This term was used by Moustakas (1994a, 1994b) to describe the filters of personal history, emotional context, and memories through which individuals frame, perceive, evaluate and respond to the outside world. It is the same concept that Harrow (2002) referred to as the "inscape" of the individual (p. 72).

Magic: Magic is intent-motivated and result-focused ancient practices and systems of rituals and activities utilizing energy to modify or manifest something in the material world (VandenBos, 2015). It has been described as an ineffable force through which things manifest, and our minds perceive concepts and phenomena belonging to the realms of spirit (Bouse, 2017; James, 1902). Magic has survived into contemporary times as an "underground esoteric tradition" (VandenBos, 2015, p. 617), and has enjoyed a resurgence in some practices associated with the New Age Movement and Neo-paganism.

Mysticism: On the one hand, mysticism is a worldview through which an individual might attain wisdom, inspiration, and revelation by means other than those of rational thought and sensory-based cognitive experience and perception. On the other hand, it is also a means through which one might connect with the "divine" (VandenBos, 2015, p. 683) in a religious context. The definition refers to states of intense, deep, and/or entranced meditations, contemplations, and ecstasies recounted in the accounts and sacred writings of global religious and spiritual traditions over time.

Neo-shamanism: Neo-shamanism is the term used for the practice of some of the ancient technologies of traditional and indigenous cultures that facilitate interaction with the spirit world for healing, divination, and sacred intervention on behalf of the community and its members by contemporary Western practitioners (Wallis, 2003). In contrast to traditional shamans who were part of magic-based, Earth-centered cultural worldviews, Neo-shamans lack such a supportive cultural matrix (Bouse, 2017). Neo-shamans frequently study shamanic techniques, e.g., journeying at will through, organizations and teaching practitioners, whereas shamans in traditional and indigenous societies are called into service by the spirit world through heredity, mystical experiences, life-threatening illness, mental crisis or near-death experience, and are trained by shamans within their communities (Eliade, 1964; Harner, 1982).

New Age: Nelson (2009) defined the New Age Movement as an emerging spirituality focused on the cultivation of the so-called inner spirit of an individual as a means of ameliorating the dissonance in one's life. Nelson explained that New Age followers believe they can connect with their so-called inner being through personal, spiritual means in order to expand their consciousness, and live more fulfilling, spiritually oriented lives.

New Religious Movement (NRM): Nelson (2009) defined a New Religious Movement as a group of individuals with common religious beliefs, which beliefs are anomalous to the beliefs embraced by the conventional organized religions of the world. Nelson further explained that some of these New Religious Movements represented a reorganization and resurgence of ancient religious beliefs and practices such as contemporary Neo-paganism and Druidism (Wallis, 2003; York, 2002).

Paranormal: Paranormal is an adjective describing the anomalous nature of activities, occurrences, observations, and manifestations that present in material reality but originate from outside of it (Colman, 2009). Similarly, VandenBos (2015) defined paranormal as being the alleged transfer of information or phenomena inexplicable by known scientific models and paradigms.

Paganism: York (2002) provided a concise definition of Paganism as an ancient system of varied religious beliefs including magic, animism, and pantheism practices by indigenous peoples and ancient tribes, including those of Europe. According to York (2002) and Wallis (2003), Neo-paganism consists of a network of loosely connected beliefs emerging from a reconstruction of alleged practices and beliefs ascribed to ancient Pagans by contemporary practitioners.

Religion: The *APA Dictionary of Psychology* (VandenBos, 2015) defines religion as a system of beliefs focused on the worship of an omnipresent deity or deities. These beliefs are expressed in standardized forms and protocols of ritual, practice and prayer. The teachings and traditions of religion are communicated through holy texts generated by sanctioned founders, philosophers, and authorities. An established religion endorses a set of moral codes backed by divine authority, and it determines which shrines, texts, and individuals are considered sacred.

Shaman: "Shaman" is the designation used to describe a spiritual or religious leader from an indigenous culture who uses "allegedly supernatural or magical powers" (VandenBos, 2015) in order to heal others and perform other sacred duties on behalf of the community through interaction with the spirit world and invocation of the powers of nature. A shaman emerges and functions in a supporting cultural matrix of beliefs and traditions and is recognized by the community as a religious or spiritual leader (Rock & Krippner, 2011).

Spirituality: The *APA Dictionary of Psychology* (VandenBos, 2015) defines spirituality as a belief system containing an implied "concern for God and a sensitivity to religious experience" (p. 1019), whether or not that sensitivity is expressed in any formal religious doctrine. Nelson (2009) expanded this definition of spirituality to include analysis and discussion of the movement of spirituality away from organized religion and towards individual seeking through religious eclecticism, including New Age spiritualities.

The *APA Dictionary of Psychology* (VandenBos, 2015) is a reliable reference for standard definition of terms within the parameters of current psychological practice. It is therefore an excellent initial resource for the definition of any terms within this book that require further clarification.

At its core *Neo-shamanism and Mental Health* is a book about the shamanic journey as an ancient mind and consciousness expanding technology that might have some surprising benefits in today's mental health context. All that is required of the reader is to keep an open mind to the possibility that we might not comprehend the totality of consciousness, and that even science has explicatory limitations.

There are more things in heaven and earth, Horatio, than are dreamt of in your philosophy. —Hamlet, *Act 1, Scene 5* (Orgel & Braunmuller, 2002, p. 1357)

References

Bouse, K. (2017). *Neo-shamanism as a developmental, spiritual matrix for contemporary magical discovery and practice* (Doctoral dissertation). Available from ProQuest Dissertations and Theses database (No. 10742675).

Colman, A. (Ed.). (2009). *Oxford dictionary of psychology* (3rd ed.). New York, NY: Oxford University Press.

Eliade, M. (1964). *Shamanism: Archaic techniques of ecstasy.* Princeton, NJ: Princeton University Press.

Harner, M. (1982). *The way of the shaman.* New York, NY: Bantam.

Harrow, J. (2002). *Spiritual mentoring: A pagan guide.* Toronto, ON, Canada: ECW.

James, W. (1902). *The varieties of religious experience.* New York, NY: Barnes & Noble.

Moustakas, C. (1994a). *Existential psychotherapy and the interpretation of dreams.* Northvale, NJ: Jason Aronson.

Moustakas, C. (1994b). *Phenomenological research methods.* Thousand Oaks, CA: Sage.

Nelson, J. (2009). *Psychology, religion, and spirituality.* New York, NY: Springer.

Rock, A., & Krippner, S. (2007). Shamanism and the confusion of consciousness with phenomenological content. *North American Journal of Psychology, 9*(3), 485–500.

Rock, A., & Krippner, S. (2011). *Demystifying shamans and their world: An interdisciplinary study.* Charlottesville, VA: Imprint Academic.

VandenBos, G. (Ed.). (2015). *APA dictionary of psychology* (2nd ed.). Washington, DC: American Psychological Association.

Wallis, R. (2003). *Shamans/neo-shamans: Ecstasy, alternative archaeologies, and contemporary paganism.* London, UK: Routledge.

York, M. (2002). *Pagan theology: Paganism as a world religion.* New York, NY: New York University Press.

Contents

List of Tables

CHAPTER 1

Contemporary Application of an Ancient Technique

Abstract This chapter examines traditional shamanism and Neo-shamanism, citing their similarities and differences. It describes the technology and process of the shamanic journey and examines its apparent ability to integrate normal waking consciousness and the executive brain with the unconscious and the limbic system. The chapter includes precautions regarding using this ancient technology without the proper instruction and/or supervision and group environment and discusses Neo-shamanism as a cultural phenomena that is anomalous to both our current cultural paradigm and academic inquiry.

Keywords Neo-shamanism · Shamanism · Shamanic journey · Cultural dissonance

> *You have no need to travel anywhere – journey within yourself.*
> *Enter a mine of rubies and bathe in the splendor of your own light.* —Rumi

The terms "shaman" and "shamanism" have come into fairly common usage over the past several decades. Shamans and their mysterious practices have been incorporated into popular culture and awareness through avenues as diverse as the academic diligence of anthropologists such as

K. J. Bouse, *Neo-shamanism and Mental Health*,
https://doi.org/10.1007/978-3-030-31911-3_1

Michael Harner and Mircea Eliade to rock 'n' roll icons such as Jim Morrison. But what exactly is shamanism? What is the nature of its practices? The idea of the shaman invokes a mystical image of an archaic and primitive (albeit powerful) sorcerer who employs an amalgam of magic, medicine, and supernormal capabilities to gain knowledge, manipulate the material world, perform miracles and healings, or exact revenge. But does the practice of shamanism potentially have any use or significance to contemporary Western societies? This small book strives to explore the phenomenon of shamanism and postulate its potential benefits if applied to our contemporary lives. The starting point of this discussion is to examine shamanism and its contemporary non-traditional counterpart Neo-shamanism in order to derive a workable definition and understanding of the terms and practices to be examined and discussed.

What Do We Mean by the Terms "Shaman" and "Shamanism?"

Shamanism is an archaic, cross-cultural spiritual technology and practice that has survived encroaching civilization, colonialism, persecution, and genocide by virtue of its preservation by remote, isolated societies (Eliade, 1964; Harner, 1982; Winkelman, 2010). Interest and awareness of shamanism emerged during the late twentieth century in the contemporary West as an alternative spirituality and healing protocol as part of the New Age movement. Its popularization was enhanced by the work of anthropologist Michael Harner through his book *The Way of the Shaman* (1982) and subsequent instructional workshops, which introduced shamanism and the shamanic journey technique to eager audiences desiring spiritual alternatives to the dominant Western religious traditions. These contemporary Western practitioners came to be designated as Neo-shamans. For Neo-shamans, the application of shamanic technique and the interpretation of the accompanying phenomena are defined by the personal meaning-making lenses and cultural matrices of individual practitioners who are not members of a culture or society that includes such practices and phenomena in its dominant paradigm. It is this lack of supporting cultural framework for shamanic practice, dissonance of cultural worldview, and absence of culturally accepted interpretative models from which to derive meaning from anomalous phenomena that differentiate contemporary Neo-shamans from shamans of the ancient past or those currently active in traditional societies.

What Is Traditional Shamanism?

Shamanism is a practice and mastery of a set of spiritual technologies which originated from archaic and indigenous cultures as a means of interacting with non-linear, ineffable powers for the purpose of benefitting the community and its members (Rock & Krippner, 2011). Such cultures are characterized by their embrace of a worldview that is animistic, pantheistic, Earth-and-nature-centered, and magic-based. It is a system of belief and *Dasein* rooted in belief in the immanent nature of divinity and the presence of the sacred in all things (Eliade, 1964; Rock & Krippner, 2011; Winkelman, 2004, 2009, 2010; Winkelman & Baker, 2010; York, 2002, 2005b). Shamanism emerged from the need of ancient peoples to create a means by which the power of divinity, as expressed in nature, might be invoked and used for the benefit of the tribe(s) for healing, divination, location of food, and protection (Campbell, 1959; Eliade, 1964; McClenon, 2011; Sala, 2014; Sarasola, 2015; Sidky, 2010; Winkelman, 2004, 2009, 2010, 2011b; Winkelman & Baker, 2010). Shamanism is a global phenomenon that has appeared throughout human history, and always with elements of the anomalous, the mythic, magic, and the transpersonal consistently present albeit with the meaning of the phenomena being subject to culturally specific interpretations (Herbert, 2011; Hunt, 2010; Malan, 2016; St. John, 2011).

The technologies used by shamans enable them to enter altered states of consciousness in order to perceive variant phenomenological patterns at will for the specific purpose of interceding with the spirit world for the benefit of the community (Krippner, 2000; Rock & Krippner, 2011; Winkelman, 2004, 2013a, 2013b). Reaching the required altered state frequently requires the use of drugs, dreams, sleep, food and sensory deprivation, and/or drumming so that the divine phenomena might be perceived (Rock & Krippner, 2007b). Through this means, the power of divinity expressed in the natural world might be invoked, approached, and solicited to effect healing, find food, divine, protect, help the dead to depart, and the newly born to enter this life with purpose and identity (Campbell, 1959; Eliade, 1964; McClenon, 2011; Sala, 2014; Sarasola, 2015; Sidky, 2010). The shaman was the tribe's liaison to the spirit world, a skilled technician who possessed the ability to traverse the material boundaries of time and space to interact with nature spirits, animal spirits, ancestors, spirit teachers, and the deceased to enlist their aid and advice for the tribe and its members, as well as do battle with malefic entities including enemy shamans and their spirit allies (Rock & Krippner, 2011; Winkelman, 2009, 2010, 2013b). Specifically induced and willed entry into an altered state of consciousness are central characteristics of shamanic practice because it is the altered state of consciousness which enables the shaman to perceive phenomena not ordinarily perceived through the process of physical sensory stimulation and subsequent cognition (Rock & Krippner, 2007b).

Shamanism is characterized by the central figure of the shaman. This is a man or a woman who has the ability to enter an altered state of consciousness at will and for a specific purpose in order to traverse time and space to perceive and confront the mythic, anomalous, magical, and transpersonal world of the divine for the benefit of the tribe or community (Rock & Krippner, 2007b; Winkelman, 2013a, 2013b). Thus, the shaman was at once physician, magician, counselor, and protector of the tribe who battled the forces threatening the community's safety and survival (Eliade, 1964; Rock & Krippner, 2011). Our current understanding of traditional shamans and shamanic practice comes predominantly through the discipline of anthropology. Scholars such as Harner and Winkelman took their academic skills into the field (sometimes at no small risk) to live among contemporary shamanic tribes in South America and Asia in order to observe the culture and the work of the shamans within it. Harner (1982) described his experiences with the Jivaro of Ecuador and the Conibo of Peru. He reported being taken on an initiatory expedition into the jungle by Conibo shamans and given Ayahuasca, which gave rise to a profound spiritual journey and near-death experience during which he was able to perceive a world far beyond that of matter. Harner's experience is consistent with research results and observations of other anthropologists like Winkelman and Eliade, gleaned from different shamanic cultures, specifically that they:

- are identified as being shamans by the tribe through experiencing of a near-death experience, serious illness, psychotic break, or receiving a waking vision or dream.
- receive training from the tribal shamans so that they can perform healing, divination, psychopomp work, and feats of *psi* such as telekinesis, distance viewing, and use of ESP.
- undergo some sort of initiation as a shaman under the direction of the tribal shaman and elders.
- frequently maintain their mundane position in the tribal society, e.g., farmer and hunter despite being recognized as one of the tribal shamans.

- frequently perceive anomalous phenomena simultaneously with physical phenomena when not in a deliberately induced altered state of consciousness.
- are dedicated to providing service to the tribe at the specific request of the tribe and its members.
- are intimately and continually connected to the world of nature and spirit.

The ancient shamans were the original psychonauts, and their descendents continue to operate traditionally within indigenous societies today.

While the technologies of shamanism and the perception of anomalous phenomena during the periods of expanded, non-waking consciousness (referred to as the shamanic journey) are cross-culturally consistent (Winkelman, 2013b), the interpretation of those phenomena varies widely based on the culture and society in which the shamanic practice is occurring. Encounters with non-material phenomena are not exclusive to shamanic societies and practice. Reports of human interactions with anomalous, spiritually based phenomena, and perceptions appear within the frameworks of contemporary world religious literatures. Ezekiel's vision of the wheel, Paul's vision of Christ on the road to Damascus, and the Marian apparitions that reportedly occurred at Lourdes, Fatima, Guadalupe, and Medjugore (Geels, 2011; Zimdars-Schwartz, 1991) are examples of perception of other-worldly phenomena recorded in the Christian tradition and interpreted within its framework of beliefs. These records of encounters with anomalous phenomena frequently report a shift of consciousness away from the mundane on the part of the perceiver. Paul's seizure and blindness, Ezekiel's visionary state (Harrelson, 2003), and the reported shifting of perception and presence of anomalous phenomena such as a spinning sun and the smell of roses described by witnesses of some of the Marian apparitions (Zimdars-Schwartz, 1991) all describe a shift away from ordinary waking consciousness into some kind of altered, hypnotic state. The deviation between the parameters and matrices of religious belief of the perceiver and those embraced by the perceiver's cultural-societal matrix frequently determine the difference between a visionary experience and a psychotic episode (Hood, Hill, & Spilka, 2009; Lukoff, 2011; Zimdars-Schwartz, 1991).

Shamanic Navigation of Consciousness

Lying at the core of any shamanic practice is the ability to shift from ordinary waking consciousness to other areas of consciousness at will and for a specific purpose (Harner, 1982; Rock & Krippner, 2011; Winkelman, 2004, 2009, 2010; Winkelman & Baker, 2010). Winkelman (2011a, 2011b) acknowledged that the phenomenon of soul flight (as related to out-of-body experiences or alteration of conscious perception from the mundane to the transpersonal) is a common denominator across all shamanic practices cross-culturally. But how does this shift in consciousness occur? Any attempt to comprehend the mechanics of the shamanic journey requires examination of some current psychological research into the nature of consciousness.

Rock and Krippner's (2007a, 2007b) research determined that so-called altered states of consciousness were variants of normal waking consciousness (Revonsuo's [2009b] normal states of consciousness) in which an individual was able to perceive different phenomenological images and patterns from those perceived in the waking state. According to Rock and Krippner (2007a), most researchers confuse consciousness with content referring to this as the "consciousness/content fallacy" (p. 33), in which the phenomenological content perceived in a specific state of consciousness was erroneously presumed to be the state of consciousness itself. This particularly applied in studies of shamanism, which is dependent on the perception and interpretation of non-waking phenomena as the foundation of an individual's lifeworld and meaning. Rock and Krippner (2007b) suggested that the term "shamanic patterns of phenomenological properties" (p. 485) replace the term *shamanic state of consciousness* used by Harner (1982) to circumvent the consciousness/content fallacy. This is an important distinction, particularly since many Neo-shamans refer to their journeys with the implication that they were traveling from Point A to Point B, in accordance with Harner's framework (1982). From an anthropological standpoint, the concept of a journey to achieve altered or shamanic states of consciousness and meet with spiritual entities may be valid and descriptive (Eliade, 1964; Harner, 1982, 2014). It would be consistent with the anthropological backgrounds of both these scholars. However, from a standpoint of psychological research, which can operate from a more traditional scientific model of observable phenomena, the distinction between content and consciousness is significant in establishing the scientific framework for research.

Adjusting consciousness at will in order to perceive particular phenomenological patterns is a cross-cultural characteristic of the shamanic experiences (Winkelman, 2011a). Yet the patterns we perceive vary, as consciousness fluctuates through the waking and sleep cycles, many of which have a biological genesis (Kokoszka & Wallace, 2011). Creative flow (Csikszentmihalyi, 1996; Linton, 2015), ingestion of psychoactive drugs (Luke, 2012), and emotional stress (Cardena, 2011) all have the potential to create variance in normal waking consciousness as well as in dream material. Psychological researchers have observed and analyzed consciousness variations using electrophysiological and neuroimaging protocols (Gawryluk, D'Arcy, Connolly, & Weaver, 2010) in an attempt to determine the biological basis of consciousness. Other psychologists have studied the effect of disorganized attachment on consciousness (Granqvist, Hagekull, & Ivarsson, 2012) and concluded that disorganized attachment had a direct correlation with mystical experiences. Experiments to determine the level of anxiety mediated by absorption of highly sensitive individuals during 45 minutes in a sensory isolation flotation tank likewise demonstrated a positive correlation between the degree of sensitivity and the frequency of mystical experiences while in the tank (Jonsson, Grim, & Kjellgren, 2014). Concurrent experiments led to the postulation that consciousness was a product of psychobiology, and variances in consciousness were dependent on metabolic, chemical, and structural factors (Vaitl, Birbaumer, Gruzelier, Jamieson, & Kotchoubey, 2013). These experiments represent attempts to determine the cause of reported perceptions of anomalous phenomena and experiences within the context and parameters of accepted psychological theories and lab-based scientific practices.

What Is Neo-shamanism?

Neo-shamanism is a contemporary Western interpretative practice of traditional shamanism by Westerners, including the belief in mysticism, anomalous phenomena, and magic. Its worldview is similar to traditional shamanic cultures in that it is animistic, pantheistic, Earth/nature-centered, and magic-based. It rests on a foundation of immanent divinity and the presence of the sacred in all things (Eliade, 1964; Rock & Krippner, 2011; Winkelman, 2004, 2009, 2010; Winkelman & Baker, 2010; York, 2002, 2005b). Neo-shamanism emerged in the 1980s as an alternative spirituality and healing protocol during the New Age movement. The publication of Michael Harner's *The Way of the Shaman* (1982) and his subsequent workshops made the traditional shamanic technique of using repetitive drumming to enter a state of consciousness different from ordinary waking consciousness accessible to contemporary Western students (DuBois, 2011; Wallis, 2003).

Shamanic practices ignited the imaginations and interest of contemporary Westerners through the alternative spirituality and healing paths of the New Age movement that arose in the West during the late twentieth century. Contemporary shamanic practitioners differ from their indigenous and ancient counterparts in two significant ways:

1. They are not native to a traditional shamanic culture. They are products of contemporary, Western culture with its focus on the exclusive veracity of materialism, rationality, and positivism.
2. They do not generally live in communities that have adopted the animistic shamanic worldview that they might serve (Wallis, 2003). Whereas traditional shamans work within communities and cultures that believe in the reality of phenomena beyond the physical senses, contemporary "Neo-shamans" lack the communities and cultural context to support their worldviews and practices (Krippner & Friedman, 2010). They therefore exist in a perpetual state of cultural dissonance (Bouse, 2017) (Table 1.1).

Table 1.1 Differences between traditional shamans and Neo-shamans

Native of shamanic culture	*Yes*	*No*
Near-death experience as call to service	Yes	Sometimes
Experiences psychotic break	Sometimes	Sometimes
Culture supports shamanic worldview	Yes	No
Trained by tribal shaman	Yes	Sometimes
Culture validates the dreamtime	Yes	No
Culture validates spiritual healing	Yes	Sometimes
Trained through non-tribal protocols	No	Yes
Recognized as shaman by society	Yes	No
Shamans in ancestry	Sometimes/Known	Sometimes/Unknown
Culture recognizes shamanic practices	Yes	No
Undergoes initiation as shaman	Yes	Sometimes
Societal belief in magic	Yes	No
Sacred, ritualistic drug use	Yes	No
Experiences cultural dissonance	No	Yes

Description of the Shamanic Journey

Worldviews and practices of Neo-shamans may include cultural and perceptual deviations from those of traditional shamans, but all shamanic practitioners undertake the shamanic journey. The shamanic journey itself is an altered state of consciousness in which the shaman encounters non-material entities in response to a focused quest to acquire healing, insight, and meaning-making information for the members of his/her tribe or community. The shamanic journey has characteristics that differentiate it from other altered states of consciousness in which anomalous phenomena might be encountered such as dreams (including lucid dreams), near-death experiences, meditations, ingestion of psychoactive drugs such as Ayahuasca and other DMT-based hallucinogens or LSD, psychotic episode, or spontaneous spiritual peak experiences.

The following are characteristics of the process of Neo-shamanic journeying as accrued through reports (Bouse, 2017; Harner, 2014) and observation by the author:

1. The journey is undertaken at for a specific purpose at the request and for the benefit of the social group or a member of it for healing, understanding, divination, or guidance.
2. The Neo-shaman embarks on this journey at a time and place of his or her own determination and with a specific purpose firmly in mind.
3. The focus of the journey is sharpened through careful articulation of the question asked or information sought after. Repetition of that question several times before the drumming begins is a useful tool for setting the focus of the journey.
4. The practitioner sets the destination of the journey and uses a predetermined route to get there.
5. The journey is frequently the core of a sacred ritual performed by the Neo-shaman that can be enhanced by community participation through drumming, music, chanting, and dancing. In all cases, the rituals are focused on the purpose of the journey and support the Neo-shaman's work.
6. The journey is the movement of conscious awareness by the practitioner through an altered state of consciousness, similar to hypnogogic or early phases of sleep in which material stimuli are removed to reveal a world imperceptible with the ordinary physical senses.

7. The journey is driven and maintained through use of a device that alters the brain activity of the practitioner. This device can be drumming, chanting, intoxication, deprivation, or dancing. Contemporary Neo-shamans frequently use steady, repetitive drumming to alter their brain activity for the duration of the journey. The combination of mild sensory deprivation (quiet environment except for drumming and dimmed lights or blindfolds) removes practitioners from the waking Alpha wave state and into a mild altered state of consciousness similar to hypnogogic or Stage One sleep. In this state, they are able to spontaneously perceive phenomena usually imperceptible during normal, waking consciousness (Harner, 1982, 2005; Rock & Krippner, 2007b).
8. The practitioner understands that their role is one of a facilitator and envoy to invoke the wisdom and assistance of spirit entities inhabiting the worlds to which they journey for healing and wisdom.
9. The practitioner remains rational and lucid throughout the journey and drives the journey through focus on specific purpose.
10. The Neo-shaman has experience and training in the journey protocol and is assisted by spirit allies in the form of plant and animal spirits, ancestral spirits, and spirit teachers. The practitioner may navigate the journey in an enhanced version of his or her normal physical form.
11. The journey is concluded once the practitioner has achieved the purpose of the journey, released the assisting spirits, and resumed normal physical consciousness. Most journeys are seven to twenty minutes in duration. To signal the end of the journey, the drumbeat becomes sporadic and then very rapid to elicit the production of Alpha waves and return the journeyer to their normal waking state.
12. All journeys are entered from a waking state and at the free will of the person undertaking the journey.

Caveats

At first glance, a shamanic journey might appear to be a relatively safe and harmless exercise, but it is not something that should be undertaken lightly and without previous training and supervision by an experienced and qualified teacher or psychotherapist. As a tool for exploring usually unperceived areas of consciousness, the shamanic journey opens the practitioner's awareness of phenomena that are supernormal and frequently anomalous in nature. The journey takes place in a state of consciousness in which people are highly receptive and operating without the usual cognitive boundaries and rationalism of normal waking consciousness. Such conditions can make people in the journey state vulnerable to potentially frightening and/or disorienting stimuli similar to those encountered in nightmares. These are experiences that have the potential to generate fear responses (Revensuo, 2009a, 2009b) and trigger traumatic memories.

Challenges in the Academic Study of Neo-shamanism

Neo-shamanism is problematic for scholars to define because it has removed the spiritual techniques of indigenous shamanic societies from their cultures of origin and transplanted them onto a set of cultural constructs that are alien to their native matrices (Rock & Krippner, 2011). The magical element present in both Neo-shamanism and traditional shamanism exacerbates research difficulties because it lies beyond the realm of modern thinking. Rock and Krippner noted that much of the so-called journey experiences of Neo-shamans incorporated a large element of fantasy albeit devoid of the darker elements which are part and parcel of shamanic practice (2008a, 2008b, 2008c). This observation is verified in the transcripts of recorded journeys by Neo-shamans (Bouse, 2017; Harner, 2014) which consistently describe similar phenomenological elements characterized by benevolence, self-focus, and fantasies reflective of the cultural context of the twenty-first-century United States and the New Age movement. This observation is consistent with those of Rock (2006), Rock and Casey (2005), and Rock, Casey and Baynes (2006) which noted the predominance of positive contemporary Western cultural imagery in the phenomena perceived by participants in the journey state. Likewise, Crockford (2011) observed the dominance of Western culture, philosophy, mythology, and theological orientation in the reported images perceived by contemporary North American Neo-shamans during their journeys. Crockford particularly noted the Abrahamic and Zoroastrian concepts of dark vs. light and good vs. evil as dominant themes in journeys by Western practitioners along with a wealth of phenomena that could be categorized as cross-cultural. He observed that occurrences of cross-cultural imagery were interpreted by the participants in his research within frameworks consistent with Western cultural constructs. Conversely, Mayer (2013) reported that in his studies, the phenomena described by German-speaking Neo-shamanic practitioners revealed a greater level of comfort with cultural dissonance to Western cultural paradigms than that of English-speaking participants as well as a greater incidence of heuristic flexibility when cross-cultural phenomena were encountered.

The presence of images from non-Western cultures, particularly those alleged to be of indigenous or archaic origin, is problematic to the qualitative study of Neo-shamanism because of the possibility that they are the result of cultural appropriation by the practitioner on some level. The strongest argument supporting such cultural appropriation rests in the perception that Neo-shamanism itself is an example of contemporary North Americans of European descent encroaching on the sacred practices and beliefs of Native Americans, interpreting them within their own cultural framework, and finally subjecting them to the mass consumerism which characterized some New Age practices (Aldred, 2000; Harner, 2014).

The opposite would appear to be true among Neo-shamanic practitioners in Europe, where the shamanic techniques are used as a means of connecting with their tribal roots (Mayer, 2013; Strmiska, 2004; Whisker, 2013). The reconnection with a tangible tribal past in Europe is also a strong element in the Neo-shamanic practices undertaken by individuals who are part of the contemporary European Pagan movement (Morgaine, 2013; Wallis, 2003). Morgaine cited the attempt of European Pagans to bridge the spiritual void caused by the Reformation and Enlightenment that denuded religion of its mysticism and removed the last societal remnants of magic from the lifeworld of Europeans during the seventeenth and eighteenth centuries. Such contemporary European Neo-shamans are part of a Reclaiming Movement focused on the rediscovery of lost ethnic and tribal traditions and identities (Morgaine, 2013). Rather than attempting to institute a globalized transpersonal spirituality (Hunt, 2010), the Reclaiming Movement views Neo-shamanism as a valuable technique by which modern Europeans (including North Americans and Australians) might reconnect with their lost cultural identities, spiritualities, folklore, mythology, and magical traditions (Luhrmann, 2012).

The Anomalous Nature of Neo-shamanism

The current literature revealed a dangling debate as to the essence of Neo-shamanism and its place and meaning within the current global, human matrix. As a result, there are arguments on both sides regarding the authenticity and efficacy of Neo-shamanic practice. The dearth of comprehensive phenomenological research leaves vast gaps in the current knowledge about the practice, thus making it difficult for researchers of Neo-shamanism to establish a baseline to serve as an anchor for research. Phenomenological analysis of Neo-shamans during journey experiences might serve to reinforce McClenon's theory (2011) that shamanic practice is a controlled expression of the genes that present as schizotypy in the general population. McClenon framed his analysis of shamanism in general within the discipline of evolutionary psychology as did Stevens and Price (2006) and Winkelman (2004). The neuroscientific studies cited by Winkelman were significant because they revealed that there are specific brain functions active during shamanic journeys that appear to produce a unique communication between the limbic system and the cerebral cortex (2010). Both Winkelman and McClenon made reference to the focus and willed change of consciousness from ordinary waking consciousness to a state in which non-ordinary phenomena might be perceived (Rock & Krippner, 2007b) and which separates shamanic experiences from the involuntary and unfocused phenomenal perception experienced by people in the throes of schizophrenic episodes (Grof, 2006; Lukoff, 2011).

The cross-cultural and trans-temporal aspects of such studies necessarily demand interdisciplinary research if Neo-shamanism is to be explored as the multi-faceted and anomalous cultural and psychological phenomenon that it appears to be. The potential for Neo-shamanic practice to act as a means by which global ecological healing might occur (Llamazares, 2015), and through which the link between the human and the spiritual might be re-defined (Sarasola, 2015) renders its practice (and practitioners) defiant of the categorizations imposed by the parameters of independent academic disciplines. Part of the anomalous and indefinable aspect of Neo-shamanism from the context of standard academic paradigms is its status as a relatively recent religio-cultural occurrence that remains to be recognized as a viable part of the spiritual schema of contemporary Westerners. Research into Neo-shamans in Brazil by Langdon and Santana De Rose (2012) concurred with the concept that Neo-shamanism is evolutionary in nature as evidenced by its cross-cultural and eclectic practices among people of dissimilar and non-indigenous societal matrices. Their research caused them to recommend that Neo-shamanism would benefit from recognition as a *Dasein* independent from other movements and philosophies by academics and scientists so that its potential to heal and reclaim the sacred might become its identifying characteristics.

Neo-shamanism as a Cultural Phenomenon

Neo-shamanism emerged from the point of intersection of the New Age movement, New Religious Movements, Neo-paganism, and Wicca (Wallis, 2003). As a revised archaic spiritual technique, Neo-shamanism allowed contemporary Westerners to modify their consciousness through means of outside stimulation to obtain the aid of the spirit world for healing, divination, and assistance with dying (Harner, 1982; Rock & Krippner, 2011). It is a protocol based on ancient tribal traditions (Campbell, 1959; Eliade, 1964), but which has been re-packaged for accessibility by contemporary spiritual consumers (Aldred, 2000; Harner, 1982). Further it is based on magic, which is a dissonant concept to the current twenty-first-century Western cultural matrix. The dominant culture of the United States has been one of integration and assimilation of a multitude of cultural traditions, including music, food, stories, and religions. Observed within this framework, Neo-shamanism represents an example of both the appropriation of Native American spirituality for profit (Aldred, 2000) and the American paradigm of cultural inclusion. Neo-shamanism became a desirable spiritual commodity when it merged with the individual spirituality-seeking wave that was the signature characteristic of the New Age movement (Amarasingarn, 2009; Bird, 2005; Fiere & Kirbis, 2009a, 2009b; Mears, 2000; Tucker, 2002). The assimilation and commercialization of diversified cultures in the United States have proven to be a lucrative element of the American business model; in this framework, anything of a spiritual or religious nature is as marketable as egg rolls or pizza (Harris, 1979). Unfortunately, application of the spirituality-for-profit model seriously undermines the sacred and spiritual viability of Neo-shamanism.

Shamanism as a technique was introduced to the educated post-counterculture seekers of alternative spiritualities who generated the New Age marketplace. It emerged as a viable path toward integrated fulfillment of body, mind, and spirit (Tucker, 2002; Versluis, 2014). It was attractive not only to New Agers, but was particularly harmonious with the beliefs of Neo-pagans and Wiccans in the United States and Europe due to its foundations in nature and magic (Bartolini, Chris, MacKian, & Pile, 2013; Berger, 2005; Langdon & Santana De Rose, 2012; Llamazares, 2015; Luhrmann, 2012; Wallis, 2003; Whisker, 2013; York, 2002, 2005a, 2005b). As such, Neo-shamanism found adherents in all of the above spiritually based subcultures that embraced it as an intrinsic part of their inherent core beliefs (Eskenazi, 2010; Wallis, 2003). This was particularly true of the Neo-pagans in

Europe who discovered shamanic aspects of their own lost [tribal and] magical traditions (Hutton, 2011; Jones & Krippner, 2012; Llamazares, 2015; Morgaine, 2013; Saunders, 2012; White, 2014; Wallis, 2003; York, 2002, 2005b).

What Aldred (2000) described as cultural larceny and exploitation of Native American spirituality by American Neo-shamans arose from the lack of an immediately observable tangible framework of European tribal models of the sacred (York, 2002). Elements of Native American spirituality such as animism, belief in a vibrant immanent and interested spirit realm, reverence for the Earth and all of nature, immanent divinity, and magic resonated with Neo-shamans (Harner, 1982; York, 2002, 2005b). It was adherence to these principles of Native American spirituality that informed Neo-shamanism's anomalous stance to the prevailing culture in the United States (Clifton, 2003; Llamazares, 2015; Mayer, 2013; Morgaine, 2013; Sarasola, 2015; Sutton, 2010; Whisker, 2013).

The dominant cultural paradigm of the United States is based in Newtonian positivism that denounced the viability of anything that was neither observable, measurable, nor predictive. Post-Reformation Christianity (which formed the bedrock of American culture) emphasized separation of humanity from the Earth and negation of mysticism and magic (Thomas, 1971). The spiritual concepts and worldviews implicit in Native American spirituality, Neo-paganism, and Neo-shamanism are in polar opposition to the dominant contemporary American (and Western) cultural paradigm (Bird, 2005; Harris, 1979; Rock & Krippner, 2011). Such an anomalous worldview as that held by Neo-shamans could easily be marginalized as naïve, primitive, and therefore negligible by the dominant culture (York, 2002). There is a fundamental dissonance between lifeworlds that perceive the sacred to be omnipresent, acknowledge magic, and accept the unseen as real, and those that believe in an omnipotent, transcendent creator God, and a reality limited to phenomena experienced through the physical senses (Hood et al., 2009; Hunt, 2010; Mayer, 2013, Morgaine, 2013; Wallis, 2003; Weston, 2011; York, 2002).

The dissonance between the Neo-shamanic worldview and that of the dominant culture of the contemporary United States caused Neo-shamanic practitioners to gravitate toward sympathetically anomalous groups such as Neo-pagans and Wiccans for community and spiritual support (Berger, 2005; Crockford, 2011; Hutton, 2011; Jones & Krippner, 2012; Luhrmann, 2012; Saunders, 2012; Starhawk, 1979; Wallis, 2003; White, 2010; York, 2005b). These groups have provided Neo-shamanic practitioners in the United States with a resonant contemporary community and spiritually harmonious matrix (DuBois, 2011; Magliocco, 2004; Mitchell et al., 2013).

Conclusions

Based on the literature, Neo-shamanism is a magic-based technique connecting contemporary anomalous practices of interfacing with the spirit world in mystical and magical contexts to the archaic past from which traditional shamanism originated (Winkelman & Baker, 2010). Contemporary practitioners frequently hold spiritual beliefs that are anomalous to that of the dominant Western culture. The beliefs and anomalous experiences that can occur during shamanic journeys are likely to influence the overall lifeworld of the practitioners. This creates a matrix conducive to the incorporation of magical practice, particularly in the area of healing, enhanced mysticism, and perception of anomalous phenomena (Bouse, 2017; Krippner & Achterberg, 2014; McClenon, 1997; Sala, 2014; Winkelman, 2010).

Despite the lack of a supportive cultural matrix in contemporary Western societies, practicing Neo-shamans has used shamanic journey technology to expand their consciousness, reconnect with forgotten tribal elements lost to colonialism, rationalism, and materialism, and to re-establish a strong relationship with the natural world and the concept of the presence of the sacred in all things. However, it is the interpretative void and dearth of structured developmental guidance created by the lack of a supportive cultural matrix that Neo-shamanic practitioners must struggle to overcome if they desire their practice to be grounded, sound, and ultimately conducive to the service of others.

The practice of Neo-shamanism and incorporation of its intrinsic culturally dissonant worldview and beliefs can create the need for practitioners to exercise caution and discretion when interacting with others who operate comfortably within the dominant cultural matrix. Therefore, the lifeworlds of Neo-shamanic practitioners are not readily revealed, discussed, or considered in academic, scientific, and therapeutic arenas. Such inclusion would require that more becomes known about Neo-shamanism, its impact on its practitioners, and its potential benefit as a tool for therapists and consciousness studies. The following chapter is an account of a research study made by the author in 2017 specifically to delve more deeply into Neo-shamanic practices and beliefs and the lifeworlds inhabited by its practitioners. The information gleaned from this study illuminated the lifeworlds of the Neo-shamanic practitioners who acted as participants. Further, it opened the doors to further inquiry and introduced the concept that the Neo-shamanic journey technology could be a valuable tool for consciousness studies, personal self-discovery, and psychotherapy.

References

Aldred, L. (2000). Plastic shamans and Astroturf sun dances: New age commercialization of Native American spirituality. *American Indian Quarterly, 24*(3), 329–352.

Amarasingarn, A. (2009). New age spirituality, quantum mysticism and self-psychology: Changing ourselves from the inside out. *Mental Health, Religion & Culture, 12*(3), 277–287.

Bartolini, N., Chris, R., MacKian, S., & Pile, S. (2013). Psychics, crystals, candels, and cauldrons: Alternative spiritualities and the question of their esoteric economics. *Social & Cultural Geography, 14*(4), 367–388.

Berger, H. (2005). Witchcraft and neo-paganism. In H. Berger (Ed.), *Witchcraft and magic: Contemporary North America* (pp. 28–54). Philadelphia, PA: University of Pennsylvania Press.

Bird, E. (2005). Going native or going naïve? Shamanism and the neo-noble savage. *Great Plains Quarterly, 25*(1), 60.

Bouse, K. (2017). *Neo-shamanism as a developmental, spiritual matrix for contemporary magical discovery and practice* (Doctoral dissertation). Available from ProQuest Dissertations and Theses database (No. 10742675).

Campbell, J. (1959). *Primitive mythology: The masks of God* (Vol. 1). New York, NY: Penguin.

Cardena, E. (2011). Altered consciousness in emotion and psychopathology. In E. Cardena & M. Winkelman (Eds.), *Altering consciousness: Multidisciplinary perspectives, vol. 2: Biological and psychological perspectives* (pp. 279–300). Santa Barbara, CA: Praeger.

Clifton, C. (2003). Smokey and the sacred: Nature, religion, civil religion and American Paganism. *Ecotheology, 8*(1), 50–60.

Crockford, S. (2011). Entering the crack between the worlds: Symbolism in Western shamanism. *The Pomegranate, 13*(2), 184–204.

Csikszentmihalyi, M. (1996). *Creativity: The psychology of discovery and invention*. New York, NY: Harper Perennial.

DuBois, T. (2011). Trends in contemporary research on shamanism. *Numen, 58,* 100–128.

Eliade, M. (1964). *Shamanism: Archaic techniques of ecstasy*. Princeton, NJ: Princeton University Press.

Eskenazi, E. (2010). *The roots of new age spirituality in United States social history* (Doctoral dissertation). Available from ProQuest Dissertations and Theses Global (UMI No. 88897031).
Fiere, S., & Kirbis, A. (2009a). New age is not inimical to religion and traditionalism. *Journal for the Scientific Study of Religion, 48*(1), 161–169.
Fiere, S., & Kirbis, A. (2009b). New age, religiosity, and traditionalism: A cross-cultural comparison. *Journal for the Scientific Study of Religion, 48*(1), 179–184.
Gawryluk, J., D'Arcy, R., Connolly, J., & Weaver, D. (2010). Improving the clinical assessment of consciousness with advances in electrophysiological and neuroimaging techniques. *BMC Neurology, 10,* 1–7.
Geels, A. (2011). Altered consciousness in religion. In E. Cardena & M. Winkelman (Eds.), *Altering consciousness: Multidisciplinary perspectives, vol. 1: History, culture and the humanities* (pp. 255–276). Santa Barbara, CA: Praeger.
Granqvist, P., Hagekull, B., & Ivarsson, T. (2012). Disorganized attachment promotes mystical experiences via a propensity for alterations in consciousness (absorption). *The International Journal for the Psychology of Religion, 22*(3), 180–197.
Grof, S. (2006). *When the impossible happens: Adventures in non-ordinary realities.* Boulder, CO: Sounds True.
Harner, M. (1982). *The way of the shaman.* New York, NY: Bantam.
Harner, M. (2005). The history and work of the Foundation for Shamanic Studies. *Shamanism (25th Anniversary Issue), 18*(1–2). Available at http://www.shamanism.org/articles/article18.html.
Harner, M. (2014). *Cave and cosmos.* Berkeley, CA: North Atlantic.
Harrelson, W. (Ed.). (2003). *The new interpreter's study Bible: New revised standard version with the Apocrypha.* Nashville, TN: Abingdon Press.
Harris, M. (1979). *Cultural materialism: The struggle for a science of culture.* New York, NY: Vintage.
Herbert, R. (2011). Reconsidering music and trance: Cross-cultural differences and cross-disciplinary perspectives. *Ethnomusicology Forum, 20*(2), 201–227.
Hood, R., Hill, P., & Spilka, B. (2009). *The psychology of religion: An empirical approach* (4th ed.). New York, NY: Guilford.
Hunt, H. (2010). Consciousness and society: Societal aspects and implications of transpersonal psychology. *International Journal of Transpersonal Studies, 29*(1), 20–30.
Hutton, R. (2011). Revisionism and counter revisionism in Pagan history. *The Pomegranate, 13*(2), 255–256.
Jones, S., & Krippner, S. (2012). *The voice of Rolling Thunder: A medicine man's wisdom for walking the red road.* Rochester, VT: Bear & Company.
Jonsson, K., Grim, K., & Kjellgren, A. (2014). Do highly sensitive persons experience more nonordinary states of consciousness during sensory isolation? *Social*

Behavior and Personality: an International Journal, 42, 1495–1506. https://doi.org/10.2224/sbp.2014.42.9.1495.

Kokoszka, A., & Wallace, B. (2011). Sleep, dreams, and other biological cycles in altered states of consciousness. In E. Cardena & M. Winkelman (Eds.), *Altering consciousness: Multidisciplinary perspectives, vol. 2: Biological and psychological perspectives* (pp. 3–20). Santa Barbara, CA: Praeger.

Krippner, S. (2000). The epistemologies and technologies of shamanic states of consciousness. *Journal of Consciousness Studies, 7,* 93–118.

Krippner, S., & Achterberg, J. (2014). Anomalous healing experiences. In E. Cardena, S. Lynn, & S. Krippner (Eds.), *Varieties of anomalous experiences: Examining the scientific evidence* (2nd ed., pp. 273–302). Washington, DC: American Psychological Association.

Krippner, S., & Friedman, H. (Eds.). (2010). *Mysterious minds: The neurobiology of psychics, mediums and other extraordinary people.* Santa Barbara, CA: Praeger.

Langdon, E., & Santana De Rose, I. (2012). (Neo)shamanic dialogues. *Nova Religio, 15*(4), 36–59.

Linton, M. (2015). Altered states of consciousness and creative expression. *International Journal of Transpersonal Studies, 34*(1–2), 98–102.

Llamazares, A. (2015). The wounded west: The healing potential of shamanism in the contemporary world. *ReVision, 23*(2&3), 6–23.

Luhrmann, T. (2012). Touching the divine: Recent research on neo-paganism and neo-shamanism. *Reviews in Anthropology, 41,* 136–150.

Luke, D. (2012). Psychoactive substances and paranormal phenomena: A comprehensive review. *International Journal of Transpersonal Studies, 31*(1), 97–156.

Lukoff, D. (2011). Visionary spirituality and mental disorders. In E. Cardena & M. Winkelman (Eds.), *Altering consciousness: Multidisciplinary perspectives, vol. 2: Biological and psychological perspectives* (pp. 301–326). Santa Barbara, CA: Praeger.

Magliocco, S. (2004). *Witching culture: Folklore and neo-paganism in America.* Philadelphia, PA: University of Pennsylvania Press.

Malan, G. (2016). Mythology, weltanschauung, symbolic universe, and states of consciousness. *Hervormde Teologiese Studies, 72*(1), 1–8.

Mayer, G. (2013). Spirituality and extraordinary experiences: Methodological remarks and some empirical findings. *Journal of Empirical Theology, 26*(2), 188–206.

McClenon, J. (1997). Shamanic healing, human evolution and the origin of religion. *Journal for the Scientific Study of Religion, 36*(3), 345–354.

McClenon, J. (2011). A community survey of psychological symptoms: Evaluating evolutionary theories regarding shamanism and schizophrenia. *Mental Health, Religion & Culture, 15*(8), 799–816.

Mears, D. (2000). Who buys new age materials? Exploring sociodemographic, religious network, and contextual correlates of new age consumption. *Sociology of Religion, 61*(3), 289–313.

Mitchell, S., Price, N., Hutton, R., Purkiss, D., Patton, K., Raudvere, C., … Sepulveda, V. (2013). Wicca and neo-paganism: A primer for counselors. *Journal of Professional Counseling: Practice, Theory and Research, 40*(1), 38–48.

Morgaine, R. (2013). The alchemy of life: Magic, anthropology and human nature in Pagan theology. *Australian Journal of Anthropology, 24*(3), 290–309.

Revonsuo, A. (2009a). Inner presence: Consciousness as a biological phenomenon. Cambridge, MA: MIT Press.

Revonsuo, A. (2009b). What is an altered state of consciousness? *Philosophical Psychology, 22*(2), 187.

Rock, A. (2006). Phenomenological analysis of experimentally induced visual mental imagery associated with shamanic journeying to the lower world. *International Journal of Transpersonal Psychology, 25*, 45–55.

Rock, A., & Casey, P. (2005). Experimental study of ostensibly shamanic journeying imagery in naïve participants I: Antecedents. *Anthropology of Consciousness, 16*(2), 72–92.

Rock, A., Casey, P., & Baynes, P. (2006). Experimental study of ostensibly shamanic journey imagery in naive participants II: Phenomenological mapping and modified effect bridge. *Anthropology of Consciousness, 17*(1), 65–83.

Rock, A., & Krippner, S. (2007a). Does the concept of "altered states of consciousness" rest on a mistake? *International Journal of Transpersonal Studies, 26*, 303–340.

Rock, A., & Krippner, S. (2007b). Shamanism and the confusion of consciousness with phenomenological content. *North American Journal of Psychology, 9*(3), 485–500.

Rock, A., & Krippner, S. (2008a). Is a realistic interpretation of shamanic non-physical worlds logically incoherent? *Transpersonal Psychology Review, 12*(2), 23–31.

Rock, A., & Krippner, S. (2008b). Proposed criteria for the necessary conditions for shamanic journeying inquiry. *Journal of Scientific Exploration, 22*(2), 215–226.

Rock, A., & Krippner, S. (2008c). Some rudimentary problems pertaining to the construction of an ontology and epistemology of shamanic journeying imagery. *International Journal of Transpersonal Psychology, 27*, 12–19.

Rock, A., & Krippner, S. (2011). *Demystifying shamans and their world: An interdisciplinary study*. Charlottesville, VA: Imprint Academic.

Sala, L. (2014). *Ritual: A magical perspective*. New Delhi, India: Nirala.

Sarasola, C. (2015). Reality, invisible world, and shamanism: An outlook from an indigenous worldview. *ReVision, 17*(2–3), 24–31.

Saunders, R. (2012). Pagan places: Towards a religiosity of neopaganism. *Progress in Human Geography, 37*(6), 786–810.

Sidky, H. (2010). On the antiquity of shamanism and its role in human religiosity. *Method & Theory in the Study of Religion, 22*(1), 68–92.

St. John, G. (2011). Spiritual technologies and altering consciousness in contemporary counterculture. In E. Cardena & M. Winkelman (Eds.), *Altering consciousness: Multidisciplinary perspectives, vol. 1: History, culture and the humanities* (pp. 203–228). Santa Barbara, CA: Praeger.

Starhawk. (1979). *The spiral dance: A rebirth of the ancient religion of the great Goddess.* New York, NY: Harper & Row.

Stevens, A., & Price, J. (2006). *Evolutionary psychology: A new beginning* (2nd ed.). New York, NY: Routledge.

Strmiska, M. (2004). Review of nine worlds of Seid-magic: Ecstasy and neo-shamanism in North European paganism by Jenny Blain. *Nova Religio, 7*(3), 99–101.

Sutton, P. (2010). Aboriginal spirituality in a new age. *Australian Journal of Anthropology, 21*(1), 71–89.

Thomas, K. (1971). *Religion and the decline of magic.* New York, NY: Charles Scribner's Sons.

Tucker, K. (2002). New age religion and the cult of the self. *Society*, January–February, 46–51.

Vaitl, D., Birbaumer, G., Gruzelier, J., Jamieson, G., & Kotchoubey, B. (2013). Psychobiology of altered states of consciousness. *Psychology of Consciousness: Theory, Research, and Practice, 1*(5), 2–47.

Versluis, A. (2014). *American gurus: From American transcendentalism to new age religion.* New York, NY: Oxford University Press.

Wallis, R. (2003). *Shamans/neo-shamans: Ecstasy, alternative archaeologies, and contemporary paganism.* London, UK: Routledge.

Weston, B. (2011). The new metaphysical: Spirituality and the American religious imagination. *Choice, 48*(5), 912–913.

Whisker, D. (2013). The possibility of shamanism: A genealogy of anthropological appropriations. *History and Anthropology, 24*(3), 344–362.

White, N. (2014). Devil's stones and midnight rites: Megaliths, folklore, and contemporary Pagan witchcraft. *Folklore, 125*, 60–79.

Winkelman, M. (2004). Shamanism as the original neurotheology. *Zygon, 39*(1), 193–217.

Winkelman, M. (2009). Shamanism and the origins of spirituality and ritual healing. *Journal for the Study of Religion, Nature & Culture, 3*(4), 458–489.

Winkelman, M. (2010). *Shamanism: A biopsychosocial paradigm of consciousness and healing* (2nd ed.). Santa Barbara, CA: Praeger.

Winkelman, M. (2011a). A paradigm for understanding altered consciousness: The integrative role of consciousness. In E. Cardena & M. Winkelman (Eds.), *Altering consciousness: Multidisciplinary perspectives, vol. I: History, culture and the humanities* (pp. 23–44). Santa Barbara, CA: Praeger.

Winkelman, M. (2011b). Shamanism and the alteration of consciousness. In E. Cardena & M. Winkelman (Eds.), *Altering consciousness: Multidisciplinary perspectives, vol. 1: History, culture and the humanities* (pp. 159–180). Santa Barbara, CA: Praeger.
Winkelman, M. (2013a). Shamanic cosmology as an evolutionary neurocognitive epistemology. *International Journal of Transpersonal Studies, 23*(1), 79–99.
Winkelman, M. (2013b). Shamanism in cross-cultural perspective. *International Journal of Transpersonal Studies, 31*(2), 79–99.
Winkelman, M., & Baker, J. (2010). *Supernatural and natural: A biocultural approach to religion*. New York, NY: Routledge.
York, M. (2002). *Pagan theology: Paganism as a world religion*. New York, NY: New York University Press.
York, M. (2005a). New age and magic. In H. Berger (Ed.), *Witchcraft and magic in contemporary North America* (pp. 8–28). Philadelphia, PA: University of Pennsylvania Press.
York, M. (2005b). Shamanism and magic. In H. Berger (Ed.), *Witchcraft and magic in contemporary North America* (pp. 81–101). Philadelphia, PA: University of Pennsylvania Press.
Zimdars-Schwartz, S. (1991). *Encountering Mary*. New York, NY: Avon.

CHAPTER 2

Method of Research

Abstract This chapter is an in-depth examination of the research method and rationale used in a 2017 study of six Neo-shamanic practitioners. The study used a mixed method of narrative, and phenomenology, and is accompanied by quantified charts and tables relevant to the results and range of participants. The discussion describing the study and its conclusions are augmented by inclusion of the research instruments (questionnaires focused on mysticism, anomalous experiences, magic, and Neo-shamanic practice and the interview template), and outline of the recorded journeys as aids to delineating the scope of the study, the means of data gathering, and as a basis for future research.

Keywords Neo-shamanic practice · Qualitative research protocol · Mysticism · Anomalous experiences · Magic

There is no need to travel anywhere. Journey within yourself. —Rumi

The inspiration and foundation for this book came from a research project that was the core of my doctoral dissertation in psychology. The dissertation, entitled *Neo-shamanism as a Developmental Spiritual Matrix for Contemporary Magical Discovery and Practice* (2017), examined the lifeworlds

K. J. Bouse, *Neo-shamanism and Mental Health*,
https://doi.org/10.1007/978-3-030-31911-3_2

of six Neo-shamanic practitioners and was directed by Drs. Stanley Krippner, Ruth Richards, and Jacquie Lewis. Each of these scholars is an acknowledged expert in their respective fields. Being an academic with thirty years experience as a Neo-shamanic practitioner, student, and teacher enabled me to conduct this study through integrated etic and emic perspectives. I approached the project from the standpoint of academic inquiry enmeshed with the personal belief that there is more to reality than what we perceive through the physical senses, that meaning-making as a personal process is frequently dependent on an individual's lenses, and that the derived meaning resulting from this process is valid. This study was successful in obtaining insight into the personal lifeworlds of Neo-shamanic practitioners, but it also revealed that the technology of the shamanic journey held promise as a data-gathering tool for consciousness and parapsychological research. It further re-enforced the concept that Neo-shamanic techniques might be useful adjuncts to therapeutic practice (Harner, 2005; McKinnon, 2012).

Overview of Research Method and Results

For purposes of academic inquiry, the research was based in peer-reviewed literature which was then followed by a qualitative, phenomenological inquiry based on six case studies for which I designed all of the protocols and instruments. The study focused on four areas of the lifeworlds of the participants that were relevant to the scope of the study. These were:

1. Mysticism,
2. Anomalous experience,
3. Magic, and
4. Neo-shamanic practice.

Each participant (a) completed questionnaires concerning their personal beliefs about each of these topics, (b) engaged in an intensive personal interview, and (c) undertook two shamanic journeys in which they simultaneously narrated the unfolding events and phenomena into a tape recorder. The research concluded that these Neo-shamanic practitioners:

- integrated aspects of indigenous, animistic cultures with their own personal histories and dominant contemporary Western culture,

- incorporated strong elements of magic and Gnosticism in their practices and worldviews,
- experienced enhanced connections to nature and spirit, a perception of consciousness beyond the material, belief in anomalous phenomena, and increased creativity,
- expressed highly personalized interpretations of the phenomena encountered in journeys to reflect their personal filters and shared cultural foundations, e.g., Christianity, and
- expressed core beliefs about mysticism, anomalous experiences, magic, and Neo-shamanic practice that were outside of the materialist/cognitive paradigm of contemporary Western culture.

A more detailed account of the 2017 study follows, including charts and reproduction of the research instruments. The methods and instruments employed in the study provide a model on which further inquiry might be based. However, it is important to note that its findings are presented as a phenomenological account without any judgment, analysis, or interpretation from the researcher.

Mixed Method: Six Case Studies and Phenomenological Analysis

Case Study Approach

According to Yin (2009), case studies are appropriate means of research for exploration, particularly when the results are the basis of information for cross-case analysis. This was especially relevant in situations in which their individual contexts and meaning-making processes influenced their interpretations of the anomalies and became incorporated into their lifeworlds.

Phenomenological Analyses

Although this was not a strict phenomenological study, the meaning of perceived phenomena and occurrences can only be determined by the experiencing individual and their assessment of its significance from within the context of their own particular lifeworld (Moustakas, 1994). The study endeavored to record accounts of the lifeworlds of the participants, which necessarily included their own interpretation of any phenomena (anomalous or otherwise) that they claimed to encounter in both normal waking consciousness and altered states (Rock & Krippner, 2007a, 2007b). This was a totally reflective exercise by the participants (Moustakas, 1994) which by its very nature is phenomenological because it excludes any interpretative or hermeneutic analysis by the researcher (Gadamer, 1975). When participants apply their own specific meaning to phenomena or set of phenomena, they supply the researcher with a sense of the deep structural meaning inherent in the participant's lifeworld (Geertz, 1973).

Research Design

The 2017 study was based on six case studies in which each participant completed three components. These components were:

- Questionnaires to determine each participant's attitude and beliefs about mysticism, anomalous experiences, magic, and Neo-shamanic practice;
- An hour long digitally recorded and transcribed interview in which the participants explored and described their personal history and lifeworlds to reveal the frequency of occurrence of phenomena and concepts which were anomalous to those of the dominant twenty-first-century American culture; and
- Two digitally recorded and transcribed 10-minute shamanic journeys focused on identical specific questions.

The data were analyzed for elements of mysticism, anomalous experiences, magic, and Neo-shamanism as they applied to the research questions. The interviews and journeys revealed elements and anecdotes that were potentially significant to this project as well as to future, deeper inquiries. All of the participants were experienced Neo-shamanic practitioners who were comfortable with undertaking journey work and sharing their experiences and interpretations. All of the participants were part of an ongoing women's spirituality and support group that self-evolved from yoga classes several years prior to this study taking place. All aspects of this study were performed in compliance with the Code of Ethics of the American Psychological Association and the US National Institutes of Health rules governing research using human participants.

Research Instruments

The research instruments—questionnaires, interview questions, and shamanic journey directives—were specifically designed to ascertain the attitudes and beliefs of the participants regarding mysticism, anomalous experiences, magic, and Neo-shamanic practice. They were designed to assess the occurrence (including nature and frequency) of perception of anomalous phenomena, and experiences, and incorporation of culturally dissonant beliefs in the individual lifeworlds, as well as their meaning to the participants within their personal contexts. Examples of anomalous phenomena might include perceiving the presence of an ancestor, a talking bird, a spirit entity, or what might appear to be an object of so-called extraterrestrial origin. All of the information elicited by the questionnaires, the interview questions, the recorded journeys, and the brief interpretative post-journey interviews helped to reconstruct the lifeworld and meaning-making lenses and processes of each participant.

The Participants

The six Neo-shamanic practitioners who were involved in this study were Euro-American females between 21 and 64 years of age who were members of a women's group that explores alternative healing protocols and spiritual pathways (Fuller, 2001) such as Reiki, shamanism, and yoga. All of them resided in an area that is predominantly rural and characterized by abundant forests, mountains, and lakes. Five of the six participants were transplants to this locale, and all but one of them has lived here for 15–25 years. Only two of the participants continued to practice any form of organized religion, with the majority having adopted varying paths of spirituality including Buddhism, New Age, and Hindu/yoga influences. One participant had completed secondary education; five have Bachelor's degrees from accredited educational institutions, and one has a Master's degree. The group reflected socioeconomic diversity: Three of the six participants grew up in blue-collar environments, one participant came from a professional background, and one participant grew up in a struggling single-parent household. Only one participant came from a privileged family. Four of the six participants reported abusive environments in their early home lives, and all of these designated the male parent as the perpetrator of the abuse.

The participants contributing to this study were unique in several ways that strengthened the validity of their responses and perceptions. These six women were dedicated to helping and healing others in ways that incorporated unconventional, alternative methods such as Reiki, Neo-shamanistic practices and protocols, and/or the use of herbs and plants for remedies. They did not consider themselves to be shamans, but rather caring practitioners who included shamanic healing techniques as part of their tool kits, strong adherence to ethical guidelines. The preservation and protection of the natural world and Mother Earth were core concerns for all of them. Each had a history of studying and practicing shamanic techniques for their own self-exploration and deep self-understanding (including facing their shadows) as well as helping others over the course of 3–8 years. Lacking a sympathetic cultural context to guide spiritual identity inclusive of shamanic practice, they believed optimal self-knowledge helped them to become clear facilitators of healing. It was their level of self-knowledge, depth of study, connection with nature and love for the Earth, and commitment to helping others that rendered their insights and personal revelations particularly valid and enriching for a study of this kind.

Table 2.1 presents a demographic overview of all of the participants showing diversities and similarities among them. More about the participants, their beliefs and practices are included in Chapter 3.

Data Gathering

Questionnaires

The data-gathering process was initiated by the participants completing four questionnaires. Each questionnaire had a specific focus.

- The Mysticism Questionnaire (Appendix 1) was designed to determine if mysticism is present in the lifeworld of the participant and, if so, what the nature and influence of such mystical beliefs are.
- The Anomalous Experiences Questionnaire (Appendix 2) was designed to determine whether the participants have had anomalous experiences, whether they believed in the veracity of them, and what the influence of any such experiences on the participant's worldview might be.
- The Magic Questionnaire (Appendix 3) sought to determine if participants believed in magic, what their definition of magic was, and how and if they used what they defined as magic in their Neo-shamanic practices and daily lives.

Table 2.1 Participant demographics

	Participant					
	1	*2*	*3*	*4*	*5*	*6*
Age	63	56	44	61	59	21
Education	Master of Business Administration	Bachelor of Arts	High School	Bachelor of Arts	Bachelor of Arts	Bachelor of Fine Arts
Occupation	Retired/Corporate	Senior Caregiver	Beautician	Yoga Instructor	Farmer	Student
Ethnicity	German/Irish	German/Irish	Scottish-Irish	German	Scottish	Scottish-Irish
Birthplace	New York	Wisconsin	South Carolina	Florida	Alabama	Tennessee
Religious tradition	Roman Catholic	Roman Catholic	Southern Baptist	Liberal Christian	Roman Catholic	Southern Baptist
Spirituality	Pagan/Christian	Christian	Southern Baptist	Buddhist/Hindu	New Age Southern Baptist	Not stated
Marital status	Married	Divorced/Single	Married	Married	Married Single	Not stated
Children	No	Yes	Yes	Yes	No	No
Tenure in shamanic practice	2.5	3.5	8	6	6	3

- The Neo-shamanic Practice Questionnaire (Appendix 4) inquired how participants defined the scope and ethics of their Neo-shamanic practice, how their individual integration of magic manifested in their practice, and how they integrated the Neo-shamanic beliefs they embraced into their overall worldviews and *Dasein*.

Any apparent redundancies in questions appearing on the Magic and Neo-shamanic Practice Questionnaires were deliberate in order to observe whether there were any inconsistencies in the answers arising from presentation of questions in slightly different contexts.

Table 2.2 illustrates the distribution of the answers given by the participants on each of the four questionnaires on a Likert scale.

The statements on the questionnaires reflected core principles and characteristic beliefs about mysticism, anomalous experience, magic, and Neo-shamanic practice. As shown in Table 2.2, all six participants' responses demonstrate Belief on the Mysticism and Neo-shamanic Practice Questionnaires. These results indicate that the participants incorporated shared perceptions and beliefs into their individual worldviews. The varied responses on the Anomalous Experiences and Magic Questionnaires demonstrated a wider range of Belief/Non-Belief concerning these subjects. Although 50% of the participants indicated Belief regarding Anomalous Experiences, one-third indicated Non-Belief, and one participant was Neutral. Likewise, half of the participants responded in the Belief category on the Magic Questionnaire, but one-third of them were Neutral, and one respondent expressed Non-Belief. These answers indicated that only half of the participants perceived anomalous experiences and magic to be integral elements of their

Table 2.2 Belief or non-belief in specific non-material phenomena

Questionnaires	*Respondent disposition*			*Total*
	Belief	*Neutral*	*Non-belief*	
Mysticism	6	0	0	6
Anomalous experience	3	1	2	6
Magic	3	2	1	6
Neo-shamanic practice	6	0	0	6

Belief = agreement or strong agreement with 51% of statements on the questionnaire; Neutral = agreement or strong agreement with 50% of statements on the questionnaire; Non-belief = disagreement or strong disagreement with 51% of statements on the questionnaire lifeworlds. The questionnaire results were consistent with the information provided by the participants in the interviews. All participants spoke of strong mystical leanings and belief in Neo-shamanic practices, but reported differing experiences, perceptions, and beliefs about anomalous experiences and magic. It is significant that none of the six participants in this study described themselves as Wiccan or Neo-pagan, and only one defined herself as New Age. They managed to successfully integrate the Christian beliefs of their upbringings with the Earth-centered worldview characteristic of the shamanic perspective, so that they were able to use shamanic technologies within a non-traditional Christian framework. A broader study which included Neo-shamanic practitioners who claimed to be Neo-pagans and/or Wiccans as participants might alter the distribution of responses.

Interviews

The second step in the data-gathering process took the form of a 1-hour interview that was digitally recorded and transcribed. The interview questions appear as Appendix 5. They were designed to allow the participants to explore and described their personal histories, lifeworlds, and beliefs in general. It was important to the validity of this study that the participants reveal the manner in which the following elements impacted the construction of their worldview and framed their interaction with the world at large. These lenses were:

- Biology/Health,
- Personal history,
- Ethnicity,
- Family,
- Collective history,
- Influence of the dominant mass-mediated culture of the contemporary United States, and
- Religious orientation.

The participants were invited to discuss their spirituality, mystical beliefs, anomalous experiences, magic, and their understanding and practice of Neo-shamanism throughout the interview. The primary focus of the interview questions was to ascertain the potential presence of these elements in their lifeworlds and to determine the extent to which their Neo-shamanic practice had impacted the prevalence and importance of these influences in their lives (if at all). The questions were designed to be reflexive and open-ended in order to provide participants with the opportunity to explore their own lifeworlds and histories. They were encouraged to reference significant experiences and phenomena (such as repeated references to hawks, wolves, or recurring dreams) that were part of their lifeworlds. Cross-references to particular phenomena occurring in both normal waking consciousness and while journeying or dreaming might indicate a permeability of boundaries separating various states of consciousness.

The interviews were deep personal narratives that illustrated the lifeworlds of these six rather exceptional women, and it is for that reason that I have chosen to include abbreviated versions of them in Chapter 3. For example, the interviews revealed that four of the six participants reported physical and/or emotional abuse toward them or their female parent in the home while they were growing up. These candid narratives offer the reader insight into the lives and lifeworlds of the women in this study and are at times stark in their detail and clarity. Both psychology and qualitative studies are about people, and it would be a disservice to the discipline and the participants to reduce their lives to charts and tables alone. However, quantification simplifies the qualitative data for readers. Table 2.3 represents the core thematic elements of the individual lifeworlds of the six participants in this study.

Table 2.3 Lifeworld themes of participants

Participant	*Interview*	*Questionnaires*	*Journeys*
1.	Celtic, mysticism, service, angels	Mysticism, Earth, magic	Water, nature, spirits
2.	Angels, saints, Jesus, divinity	Mysticism, divinity, magic	Light, angels, saints
3.	Ghosts, control, Christ, angels	Mysticism, anomalous experiences	Air, animals, ancestor
4.	Fantasy, shape shifting, spirits	Mysticism, magic, nature	Nature, energy, spirits
5.	Angels, nature, light, purpose	Mysticism, anomalous experiences	Light, purity, energy
6.	Angels, ghosts, God, nature	Mysticism, anomalous experiences	Not applicable

Shamanic Journeys and Post-journey Interview for Interpretation
The third stage of data gathering took the form of two shamanic journeys in which each participant solicited the aid of spirit entities to answer specific questions. Each journey was 10 minutes or less in length. The participant was informed of the focus of the journeys. The questions for these journeys were:

1. What can people do locally to protect the environment?
2. What might I, as a Neo-shamanic practitioner, do to help facilitate healing for someone who is suffering from severe influenza?

These questions were selected because they were relatively neutral and unlikely to elicit emotional responses from the participants.

During the journeys, the participants listened to a drumming CD through earbuds and narrated the journey phenomena into a tape recorder as the journey unfolded in real time. As they narrated the course of their journeys out loud into the recorder, I made notes to facilitate the separation of images and other occurring phenomena such as events and actions. These notes provided cues for the post-journey interview in which the participants analyzed their journeys within their own contexts and started to make meaning out of what they had experienced while in the altered state. The purposes of the post-journey interviews were to allow the participants to articulate in their own words (a) the nature of the phenomena they perceived during the journeys; (b) the meaning of the phenomena perceived according to the participants; and (c) the consistency of the context, perceived phenomena, and their meanings between normal waking consciousness described in the interviews and the world experienced during the journeys. Consistency might be indicative of expanded waking consciousness, while strong differences might indicate the presence of a non-integrated and truly anomalous aspect of total consciousness. All of the interpretative post-journey interviews were recorded.

The phenomena perceived and narrated by the participants during these journeys reflected their individual lifeworlds to a large extent. For example, the participant who had the strongest New Age spiritual orientation reported fountains of crystal and interaction with light beings. The woman whose childhood was spent in South America and the Caribbean narrated journeys that took her to an entirely fantastic world wherein boundaries were permeable; she became the dragon she saw and then became just a shape on its back, interacted directly with the virus that causes influenza and perceived its consciousness. This is a phenomenon that is not usually reported by contemporary Westerners who tend to stick more to the material, natural world, but is consistent with journey reports of traditional shamans (Eliade, 1964; Harner, 2014; Winkelman, 2010). The participant who grew up in a strong, positive Roman Catholic environment reported the presence of the Archangels Michael and Raphael in her journeys, while those who reported having corporate and business backgrounds described journey landscapes that were enhanced mirrors of Earthly places. All participant narrations revealed interactions with animal spirits. These reports raised some questions regarding boundary definition, identity limitations, and the influence of the childhood environment on individual lifeworlds, and the phenomena perceived in journeys.

Data Analysis and Reporting

The primary purpose of the data analysis was to break out the anomalous elements and phenomena incorporated in a Neo-shaman's lifeworld and to determine the presence of common elements such as mysticism, magic, and anomalous experiences across the range of participants. Secondarily, the interpretation of specific phenomena within the context of participants' individual beliefs and lifeworlds added insight into those lifeworlds and provided potential clues as to the prevalence of worldviews that are inconsistent with those of the dominant culture. For example, someone who uses Neo-shamanic practice to facilitate healing or to gather information through conversation with a deceased ancestor might subscribe to traditional Christian beliefs, albeit with a slightly mystical interpretation. Such an individual may hold a worldview that is more harmonious with the dominant culture than (for example) someone who was Wiccan and perceived the world through the context of magic.

Based on the information accumulated through the research protocol, it was possible to draw potential conclusions regarding the influence of mysticism, magic, and anomalous experiences among some current Neo-shamanic practitioners and to define the common elements in their lifeworlds and the ways in which these lifeworlds were anomalous to the dominant reality constructs of contemporary American society and culture.

Alternative Spiritualities and Cultural Dissonance

Alternative spiritualities such as New Age, Neo-paganism, Druidism, and Wicca constitute part of what are recognized by some psychologists as New Religious Movements (Hood, Hill, & Spilka, 2009; Nelson, 2009). These incorporate models of spirituality that include acknowledgment of and interaction with disembodied entities (usually imperceptible through the ordinary senses) and embraced as part of an overarching spiritual matrix that might potentially exert significant influence on an individual's lifeworld and subsequent *Dasein* (Irwin, 2009; Kripal, 2010; Smith, 2007; Winkelman & Baker, 2010). The New Age and contemporary Neo-pagan spiritualities that emerged during the twentieth century in the West have continued to draw followers away from mainstream organized religious beliefs and practices toward more individualized spiritualities, including those that are based in mysticism and magic (Wallis, 2003).

As a technique by which people might access the spirit world for healing and guidance, Neo-shamanic practice intersects multiple expressions of alternative spiritualities (McKinnon, 2012; Wallis, 2003). Despite living in lifeworlds that are anomalous to that of the dominant cultural paradigm, many people on alternative spiritual paths are able to function successfully in all aspects of contemporary Western society (McKinnon, 2012; York, 2002). They embrace personal lifeworlds that are fundamentally dissonant with contemporary Western culture which is characterized by materialism, rationalism, positivism, and a limited reality constructs dependent on sensory-perceived phenomena. The difference between such lifeworlds and those generally accepted by our contemporary Western culture as customary is the substitution of beliefs unique to the individual for those designated as legitimate by the established traditions and institutions, including the ecclesiastical authorities of organized religions (Hood et al., 2009). Neo-shamanism itself is a body of archaic techniques employed by modern practitioners that are anchored in an animistic, magical matrix characterized by alleged perception of and interaction with anomalous phenomena (Winkelman & Baker, 2010). Such characteristics are dissonant not only with the religious and scientific paradigms at the core of contemporary Western culture, but with those of science as well (Eliade, 1964; Irwin, 2009; Nelson, 2009).

Anomalous Lifeworlds and Mental Health

The 2017 research project explored the individual alternative lifeworlds of six participants who have integrated mysticism, magic, anomalous experiences, and Neo-shamanic practice into their spiritual orientations and daily lives. Despite their anomalous worldviews, these individuals appeared to continue to function successfully as parents, business people, professionals, and responsible citizens in their communities operating within the parameters of the mores of the dominant culture. The research specifically focused on the manner in which Neo-shamanic practice might provide a magic-based method of connection to unseen realms of consciousness, thus enhancing and facilitating the incorporation of mystical, alternative spirituality into the lifeworlds of the participants. It simultaneously examined the role Neo-shamanic practice might play to enhance the growth and expression of a more authentic way of being in the world than that afforded to us through adherence to a spiritual paradigm that may no longer fit one's individual needs and worldviews.

Could such a practice and associated expanded worldview possibly facilitate improved mental health for those who embraced it?

This question emerged as the research went deeper into the lifeworlds of the participants, and they revealed more about their authentic identities as opposed to the personae they used to interact with the outside world. Frequently, these authentic identities were inconsistent with the accepted norms of our society and contemporary Western cultural definitions of what constitutes "reality." Working with archangels to heal someone's fever, receiving answers to questions from animals, hearing a tree's instructions on how to help it grow, using the power of air to dissipate illness, and direct communication with a virus are generally perceived as the stuff of fantasy and science fiction rather than actual human abilities. To expound on these so-called supernatural attributes publicly would likely result in the claimant being considered "crazy" by many people who accepted the prescribed worldview of our current dominant culture. To be "crazy" carries with it a negation of one's credibility and viability as a useful member of the tribe and resultant shunning by one's fellow tribe mates (McClenon, 1997). The stories of the six participants in this study include references to the unpleasantness they experienced by revealing their authentic selves as they perceived them to be to their more conforming acquaintances.

These reports inspired more questions about the nature of authentic, non-conforming identity resulting from a transpersonal practice such as Neo-shamanism, in particular:

- How does such a practice influence one's identity?
- How might an expanded lifeworld influence one's *Dasein*?
- At what point does the need to live in the world as one's authentic self override social conditioning to conform in order to survive as a viable member of the society?

These questions arose after the completion of the research project and represent areas of further inquiry that need to be explored for greater understanding of this dynamic of change. Plumbing the anomalous lifeworlds of the six Neo-shamanic practitioners in this study incorporated these subsidiary questions:

1. How do the participants define *magic* and how do they incorporate it into their practice of Neo-shamanism?
2. How strong is the influence of mysticism in the participants' lifeworlds and how does it impact their individual *Dasein*?
3. In what ways does Neo-shamanic practice reflect the spiritual/religious matrix of the individual practitioners?

Since Neo-shamanism is itself intrinsically inconsistent with dominant contemporary Western culture, it was the intent of this study to investigate the ways through which individual practitioners integrated the anomalous aspects of their practices and beliefs into their lifeworlds in the absence of a supporting cultural matrix. The interviews, journeys, and questionnaires revealed that the process of making meaning of the phenomena encountered in journeys was dictated by personal perceptions rather than cultural paradigms.

Conclusions

The dominant culture of the contemporary United States (including the accepted religious and spiritual paradigms of this culture) provided a common matrix for all of the participants in this study. Based on their questionnaire and interview responses, and journey narratives, all of them appear to have incorporated elements of the accepted spiritual beliefs of the core culture and integrated them with resonant elements of Eastern religion and New Age philosophy, their own personal histories, and evolved individual lifeworlds from that matrix. The common denominators present in the lifeworlds of all of the participants were a strong awareness of and connection to the natural world and acknowledgment of the presence of entities and phenomena invisible to the material eye.

The study of Neo-shamanism and its practice have provided the participants with a technique for accessing realms of consciousness existing beyond the cognitive capabilities of the physical sense which facilitates their search for gnosis, and their realization of their desires for lives lived with purpose and serving others. The Gnostic aspect of the Neo-shamanic practice revealed by the women in the study is significant because each of the participants claimed that incorporating shamanic technique, worldview, and practice in their lives opened new dimensions of self-exploration through which they were able to discover previously hidden personal aspects and reform elements of their identity based on the realization of an authentic, individuated version of the self. They affirmed that it has helped them to recognize their potentials and instilled a desire in them to live for a higher purpose beyond the parameters of the dominant culture (DeConick, 2016; Segal, 1992; Smith, 2007).

The participants discussed the mysterious processes they discovered through which healing is achieved, awakening or unfolding occurs, and dreams and visions are made manifest in consensual material reality. They described this as a magical and inexplicable process and unanimously expressed belief that this process was capable of effecting change in the material world. They felt that it was of mystical and divine origin and found nothing sinister or destructive in it. Based on the comments and observed experiences of the participants, this process is something requiring further study, as are the subjects of fantasy proneness, sleep paralysis, biographical identity reconstruction, and spiritual bypassing. This study corroborated earlier findings by other psychologists cited throughout this book, although those studies were not limited to Neo-shamans. Based on the sample of participants in this study, Neo-shamanic practice offers its followers a developmental and spiritual matrix for potentially transformative self-discovery that embraces an ineffable process that these participants perceived as a form of magic within the frameworks of their individual definitions and beliefs.

Further study of the magical and Gnostic elements of Neo-shamanism using a wider base of participants would promote understanding of the potential transformative aspects such a practice might facilitate. Possible studies might include investigation of the links between shamanism and Gnosticism (DeConick, 2016), and the role of these two philosophies might play in personal discovery and alchemy (Jung, 1967, 1968; Segal, 1992; Smith, 2007). Inquiry on the role and mechanics of the magical process used by some Neo-shamanic practitioners to effect change on the material level has the potential to provide some insight into the influence of consciousness on the physical plane.

Neo-shamanism is a rich ground for exploration because it is a matrix of mysticism, anomalous experience, and magic practiced by contemporary Westerners using an ancient spiritual technique that has the potential to improve our understanding of consciousness, identity, and realization of our human potential.

In the next chapter, the reader will be able to enter into the lifeworlds of the six participants as expressed in their own words. There is a great deal to be learned from these accounts from the mental health perspective because the participants are revealing their authentic selves rather than simply presenting personae. Chapter 3 examines the mental health benefits the participants reported by virtue of living in alignment with their authentic selves, despite the ever-present element of cultural dissonance they experienced.

Appendix 1: Mysticism Questionnaire

Please Answer All Questions with the Number that Best Matches Your Response:

1. Strongly Disagree (−)
2. Disagree (−)
3. Neither Agree nor Disagree (N)
4. Agree (+)
5. Strongly Agree (+)

(+) (−) (N) indicate responses of individual participants to each statement.

( ) I believe in a single divinity. +/3, −/2, N/1
( ) I believe in angels. +/6, −/0, N/0
( ) I believe in a creator God who dwells in heaven. +/2, −/3, N/1
( ) I believe in heaven and hell. +/2, −/3, N/1
( ) I believe in the superiority of humanity over nature. +/1, −/3, N/2
( ) I believe that divinity is present in all living things. +/6, −/0, N/0
( ) I believe that animals have sentience. +/6, −/0, N/0
( ) I believe that plants have sentience. +/6, −/0, N/0
( ) I believe that stones have sentience. +/4, −/1, N/1
( ) I believe that humanity is descended from alien beings. +/1, −/1, N/4
( ) I believe in a creator Goddess. +/3, −/1, N/2
( ) I believe in multiple divinities. +/5, −/1
( ) I believe that our dreams are frequent messages from greater consciousness. +/6, −/0, N/0
( ) I believe that all beings are One. +/5, −1, N/0
( ) I believe that everything is sacred. +/5, −/1, N/0
( ) I believe that there are nature spirits (including fairies). +/6, −/0, N/0
( ) I believe in the presence of a personal God. +/5, −/1, N/0
( ) I believe that the material plane is only one aspect of total Being. +/6, −/0, N/0
( ) I believe in the existence of Satan. +/2, −/1, N/3
( ) I believe in the battle of good vs evil. +/4, −/2, N/0
( ) I believe in the power of prayer.+/6, −/0, N/0
( ) I believe that there are many things that science has to date been unable to explain. +/6, −/0, N/0
( ) I believe that science has the potential to explain more than it has to this point. +/6, −/0, N/0
( ) I believe in miracles. +/6, −/0, N/0
( ) I believe in the capability of the spirit to heal. +/6, −/0, N/0

Appendix 2: Anomalous Experiences Questionnaire

Please Answer All Questions with the Number that Best Matches Your Response.

1. Strongly Disagree (−)
2. Disagree (−)

3. Neither Agree nor Disagree (N)
4. Agree (+)
5. Strongly Agree (+)

(+) (−) (N) indicate responses of individual participants to each statement.

( ) I have had prophetic dreams. +/2, −/2, N/1
( ) I can communicate with animals telepathically. +/5, −/0, N/1
( ) I can communicate with other people telepathically. +/3, −/1, N/2
( ) I frequently experience synchronicities. +/6, −/0, N/0
( ) I have seen ghosts. +/3, −/3, N/0
( ) I have sensed the presence of unseen spirits. +/6, −/0, N/0
( ) I have encountered extraterrestrials. +/1, −/4, N/1
( ) I have seen or sensed the presence of deceased ancestors. +/5, −/1, N/0
( ) I have seen or sensed the presence of deceased loved ones whom I have known. +6, −/0, N/0
( ) I have seen animals that were not animals but shape shifters. +/3, −/2, N/1
( ) I have participated in faith healings. +/3, −/3, N/0
( ) I have felt the presence of a large beneficence. +/5, −/1, N/0
( ) I have felt the presence of malefic entities. +/5, −/1, N/0
( ) I have been saved from misfortune by the timely intervention of a spirit. +/4, −/0, N/2
( ) I have been saved from accident by the timely intervention of a spirit. +/5, −/0, N/1
( ) I have experienced spirit beings talking to me in my sleep. +/4, −/2, N/0
( ) I receive messages from unseen entities from time to time. +/4, −/0, N/2
( ) I have a strongly developed intuition. +/5, −/1, N/0
( ) I have predicted the outcome of events correctly. +/4, −/2, N/0
( ) I have seen auras around living things. +/5, −/1, N/0
( ) I am sensitive to vibratory emanations. +/4, −/2, N/0
( ) I have sensed myself to be in two places at once. +/2, −/4, N/0
( ) I see spirit entities around people. +/1, −/3, N/2
( ) I have received strong messages not to do a particular thing. +/5, −/1, N/0

( ) I have experienced a miraculous healing. +/4, −/2, N/0
( ) I have experienced being out of my body. +/3, −/2, N/1
( ) I know things before they happen. +/2, −/3, N/1
( ) I have had a near-death experience. +2, −/4, N/0

Appendix 3: Magic Questionnaire

Please Answer Each Question with the Number that Best Reflects Your Response.

1. Strongly Disagree (−)
2. Disagree (−)
3. Neither Agree nor Disagree (N)
4. Agree (+)
5. Strongly Agree (+)

(+) (−) (N) indicate responses of individual participants to each statement

( ) I believe in magic. +/5, −/0, N/1
( ) I believe that someone can change things through using magic. +/4, −/0, N/2
( ) I am what most of society would refer to as superstitious. +/1, −/2, N/3
( ) I use ritual to focus my attention on something I wish to manifest in waking consciousness. +/5, −/0, N/1
( ) I have lighted candles for prayer or meditation. +/5, −/1, N/0
( ) I believe in the power of amulets for protection. +/3, −/0, N/3
( ) I believe that there is a magical element to spiritual healing. +/6, −/0, N/0
( ) I have encountered and fought ill-intentioned spirits. +/3, −/2, N/1
( ) I have devised rituals to bring something into manifestation in my life. +/3, −/2, N/1
( ) I am able to move between worlds. +/2, −/3, N/1
( ) I am a shape shifter. +/0, −/3, N/3
( ) I speak to the spirits of the deceased. +/4, −/2, N/0
( ) I speak to the spirits of the natural world. +/6, −/0, N/0
( ) I am able to look into the minds and hearts of others. +/4, −/1, N/1

( ) I see art as a means of magical expression. +/4, −/0, N/2
( ) I have used my body to raise energy and awareness in order to strengthen an intention. +/5, −/0, N/1
( ) I believe that magic should be used only for good. +5, −/0, N/1
( ) I have invoked the intercession of nature and divine entities to influence the weather. +/3, −/1, N/2
( ) I believe that magic is energy and is there to be used. +/4, −/0, N/2
( ) I have magically blessed someone. +/3, −/0, N/3
( ) I have sought to do harm to another for revenge using magical means. +/0, −/6, N/0
( ) I have successfully brought something into material manifestation through magical practice. +/2, −/1, N/3
( ) I believe that every thought, word, and action are a magical act. +/2, −/2, N/2
( ) Magic frightens me. +/0, −/4, N/2

Appendix 4: Neo-shamanic Practice Questionnaire

Please Answer Each Question with the Number That Best Reflects Your Response.

1. Strongly Disagree (−)
2. Disagree (−)
3. Neither Agree nor Disagree (N)
4. Agree (+)
5. Strongly Agree (+)

(+) (−) (N) indicate responses of individual participants to each statement

( ) I believe that shamanic practice is a magical practice. +/6, −/0, N/0
( ) I believe that using shamanism as a means of gaining greater knowledge and insight into myself is a valid use of the journey technique. +/6, −/0, N/0
( ) I believe that using shamanism as a means of gaining greater knowledge and insight into the world is a valid use of the journey technique. +6, −/0/, N/0

( ) I believe that using shamanism as a means of gaining insight into greater consciousness is a valid use of the journey technique. +6, −/0/N/0
( ) I would only use shamanic practice to help others. +6, −/0, N/0
( ) Shamanic healing is an application of magic for the good of someone else. +/5, −/0, N/1
( ) I would use shamanic practice to further my own goals. +/4, −/1, N/1
( ) I would use shamanic practice to influence people and events outside of myself without their first requesting it. +/1, −/5, N/0
( ) I believe that shamanic practice has the power to change things on the material plane. +/6, −/0, N/0
( ) Shamanic practice is a valid means by which magic can be harnessed to help others provided they have asked for such help. +/6, −/0, N/0
( ) I understand that in undertaking shamanic practice I may be dealing with entities and forces that are far stronger than my ability to control them. +6, −/0, N/0
( ) I believe that intent of the practitioner determines whether shamanic magic is a benevolent or malevolent force. +6, −/0, N/0
( ) Mental focus is imperative in shamanic practice. +/6, −/0, N/0
( ) I understand that whatever I do by using shamanic technique for a specific purpose may have unseen repercussions for the future. +/6, −/0, N/0
( ) I work predominantly with animal spirits. +/2, −/0, N/4
( ) I ask spirit animals to accomplish the purpose of my journey. +/4, −/1, N/1
( ) I ask spirit teachers to accomplish the purpose of my journey. +/3, −/1, N/2
( ) I am the primary agent of healing. +/1, −/2, N/3
( ) I am the primary agent in divination. +/1, −/3, N/2
( ) I am the primary agent of psychopomp work. +1, −/3, N/2
( ) I believe what I learn in journeys. +6, −/0, N/0
( ) I usually journey to the Upper World. +3, −/2, N/1
( ) I usually journey to the Lower World. +/5, −/0, N/1
( ) I believe that all entities encountered in shamanic journeys are benign. +2, −/3, N/1
( ) I believe that there are malefic entities that might be encountered during a shamanic journey. +6, −/0, N/0

Appendix 5: Interview Questions

1. Tell me about your childhood and your growing up?
   (a) Did you hear many fairy tales?
   (b) Did you have any strange experiences with ghosts or fairies?
   (c) Did people around you believe in the unseen?
   (d) What was your religious upbringing like?
2. When did you begin to sense that you might see the world differently than the other people around you?
3. Was there any specific event or series of events that caused you to see the world differently? If so, in what way?
4. Did you believe in magic as a child? Did you used to talk to animals? Did you have imaginary friends? Did you believe that there was truth in fairy tales and legends?
5. What kind of movies did you see growing up?
6. Do you like sci-fi and fantasy books, movies, and TV shows?
7. Are you a video gamer?
8. How would you describe consciousness from your point of view?
9. Do you sense the presence of unseen entities around you?
10. Do you perceive neo-shamanism as a magical practice? If so, how do you incorporate magic into your practice?
11. Do you believe yourself to be psychic? If so, why?
12. Do you believe in the existence of angels? Of extraterrestrial beings?
13. How would you describe the boundaries of time and space?
14. If you were taking a walk in the woods on a beautiful summer day, how would you describe what you are experiencing?
15. Do you have a strong connection with the Earth?
16. Do you believe that you have any magical capabilities? If so, please describe.
17. Do you believe in the presence of the sacred in all things? If so, do you live your daily life within the context of this belief?
18. How do you perceive your beliefs and worldview as being different from those of most people within our society?
19. Do you have difficulty relating to many things in our culture?
20. How would you describe divinity?
21. Do you feel that you belong in this time and place?

22. How do you reconcile your worldview with that of the dominant culture in order to maintain functionality in daily life? What devices do you use to balance these two worlds?
23. How would you classify your current spiritual orientation if at all (exp. Christian, Pagan, Gnostic, Wiccan, etc.)
24. Would you describe what you see and experience in the Lower World?
25. Would you describe what you see and experience in the Upper World?
26. Do you see animal spirits and spirit teachers around you when you are not journeying?
27. Do your dreams ever reflect your journeys?
28. Do you find elements of your journeys or phenomena related to them appearing in your everyday waking life?

References

Bouse, K. (2017). *Neo-shamanism as a developmental, spiritual matrix for contemporary magical discovery and practice* (Doctoral dissertation). Available from ProQuest Dissertations and Theses database (No. 10742675).

DeConick, A. (2016). *The Gnostic new age: How a countercultural spirituality revolutionized religion from antiquity to today.* New York, NY: Columbia University Press.

Eliade, M. (1964). *Shamanism: Archaic techniques of ecstasy.* Princeton, NJ: Princeton University Press.

Fuller, R. (2001). *Spiritual but not religious: Understanding unchurched America.* New York, NY: Oxford University Press.

Gadamer, H.-G. (1975). *Truth and method.* New York, NY: Bloomsbury.

Geertz, C. (1973). *The interpretation of cultures.* New York, NY: Basic.

Harner, M. (2005). The history and work of the Foundation for Shamanic Studies. *Shamanism (25th Anniversary Issue), 18*(1–2). Available at http://www.shamanism.org/articles/article18.html.

Harner, M. (2014). *Cave and cosmos.* Berkeley, CA: North Atlantic.

Hood, R., Hill, P., & Spilka, B. (2009). *The psychology of religion: An empirical approach* (4th ed.). New York, NY: Guilford.

Irwin, H. (2009). *The psychology of paranormal belief: A researcher's handbook.* Hatfield, Hertfordshire, UK: University of Hertfordshire Press.

Jung, C. (1967). *Alchemical studies.* Princeton, NJ: Princeton University Press.

Jung, C. (1968). *Psychology and alchemy.* Princeton, NJ: Princeton University Press.

Kripal, J. (2010). *Authors of the impossible: The paranormal and the sacred*. Chicago, IL: University of Chicago Press.

McClenon, J. (1997). Shamanic healing, human evolution and the origin of religion. *Journal for the Scientific Study of Religion, 36*(3), 345–354.

McKinnon, C. (2012). *Shamanism and spirituality in therapeutic practice*. London, UK: Singing Dragon.

Moustakas, C. (1994). *Phenomenological research methods*. Thousand Oaks, CA: Sage.

Nelson, J. (2009). *Psychology, religion, and spirituality*. New York, NY: Springer.

Rock, A., & Krippner, S. (2007a). Does the concept of "altered states of consciousness" rest on a mistake? *International Journal of Transpersonal Studies, 26*, 303–340.

Rock, A., & Krippner, S. (2007b). Shamanism and the confusion of consciousness with phenomenological content. *North American Journal of Psychology, 9*(3), 485–500.

Segal, R. (1992). *The Gnostic Jung*. London, UK: Routledge.

Smith, C. (2007). *Jung and shamanism in dialogue*. New York, NY: Paulist.

Wallis, R. (2003). *Shamans/neo-shamans: Ecstasy, alternative archaeologies, and contemporary paganism*. London, UK: Routledge.

Winkelman, M. (2010). *Shamanism: A biopsychosocial paradigm of consciousness and healing* (2nd ed.). Santa Barbara, CA: Praeger.

Winkelman, M., & Baker, J. (2010). *Supernatural and natural: A biocultural approach to religion*. New York, NY: Routledge.

Yin, R. (2009). *Case study research: Design and methods* (4th ed.). Los Angeles, CA: Sage.

York, M. (2002). *Pagan theology: Paganism as a world religion*. New York, NY: New York University Press.

CHAPTER 3

Neo-shamanism as an Alternative Contemporary Worldview

Abstract This chapter is twofold in that it (1) explores the lifeworlds of the Neo-shamanic practitioners participating in the 2017 study and (2) discusses the benefits they reportedly experienced as a result of their Neo-shamanic practice. It examines the worldviews of the six study participants based on their responses to the questionnaires and the verbatim transcript of their interviews and recorded journeys. These provide an intimate look at the *Dasein* and personal identities of the participants, and how their personal histories, beliefs, and spiritual orientations are integrated and reflected in their Neo-shamanic practice and journey experiences. The chapter proceeds to examine the beneficial effects of Neo-shamanic practice reported by the participants, specifically elevated well-being, enhanced identity and *Dasein*, expanded consciousness, and integration of the mystic and the mundane realms of being.

Keywords Lifeworlds · Neo-shamanic practice · Well-being · Identity · Dasein · Expanded consciousness · Shamanic journeys

K. J. Bouse, *Neo-shamanism and Mental Health*,
https://doi.org/10.1007/978-3-030-31911-3_3

> *Beauty surrounds us, but usually we need to be walking in the garden to know it.* —Rumi

This chapter will view the ways in which Neo-shamanism has affected the lives of those who practice it. The original research project focused on the evolving beliefs of the practitioners concerning mysticism, anomalous experiences, and magic. Now it's time to investigate the ways in which Neo-shamanic practice and its accompanying worldview(s) can possibly impact one's mental health and overall well-being by encouraging changes in identity and *Dasein* more aligned with the authentic self. How have the participants integrated their expanded consciousness and revised identities with ordinary waking consciousness in order to continue functioning successfully in the mundane world? We shall specifically look at their reports that reflect improved well-being, identity re-evaluation, *Dasein*, and expanded consciousness.

Through the course of their Neo-shamanic practice, the six women in the 2017 study integrated beliefs dissonant with those of the current, materialistic culture into their daily lives. Many traditional and/or indigenous cultures embrace the mystical concepts of immanent divinity, animism, a deep connection to nature, existence of a world of spirits adjacent to the ordinary world bounded by that which can be perceived by the physical senses, the veracity of dreams and what we call anomalous experiences, and the presence of magic as core elements of their cultural matrix. Our contemporary Western culture neither encompasses nor encourages such beliefs. Rather it tends to view mysticism, anomalous experiences, and magic (including healing with the aid of the spirit world) eccentric at best and pathological at worst, as evidenced in the *DSM-V* (2013). This is especially true when the person reporting such beliefs and/or experiences is not from a recognized cultural matrix that incorporates this type of belief such as Native American or other tribal culture. Someone who has grown up within the contemporary Western culture that is defined by rationality, positivism, and the exclusive dominance of the sensory, physical world but yet holds a worldview that embraces the anomalous, animistic, magical, and miraculous elements more typical of traditional cultures is likely to be considered deviant by the mental health standards of the dominant cultural worldview. The resultant cultural dissonance has the potential to create existential dilemmas for those who must live in the contemporary, sensory-defined, and bounded world, and yet who exist in a far-reaching universe that is negated by the society's paradigms. Yet the participants here and in other reports

(Harner, 2014; McKinnon, 2012) expressed enhanced well-being derived from a closer connection to nature and spirit, and a positive re-visioned identity incorporating the newly discovered authentic self. They have opted to live their lives and exist in a lifeworld consistent with their authentic beliefs rather than attempting to adjust to a dissonant paradigm that negates the validity of their own lived experience and perception.

The reports of the participants in the 2017 research study were consistent with similar reports found in books (Harner, 2014; McKinnon, 2012) as well as those I have personally encountered in workshops and classes as both a student and teacher over the past three decades. McKinnon included an in-depth discussion of the enhanced well-being reported by some of her clients in *Shamanism and Spirituality in the Therapeutic Practice* (2012). Likewise, the six women in this study have been forthcoming in expressing their personal beliefs and anomalous experiences, as well as exposing their authentic selves. The following are excerpts from the transcribed interviews I conducted with the participants in the summer of 2017. The interviews reflect the manner in which these women have integrated their Neo-shamanic practice and its accompanying expanded worldview with their lives and identities in the mundane world. There are several recurring themes that appear in these narratives:

1. Expanded consciousness beyond the ego and the physical/material world;
2. Elevated sense of well-being;
3. Close connection with nature;
4. Belief and/or experience of anomalous phenomena;
5. Acceptance of elements of animism and magic, and an awareness of the presence of the sacred in all things;
6. Simultaneous interaction with both normal and supernormal worlds;
7. Presence of mysticism in worldview and everyday life.

The Participants

Participant 1 (DG)

This is a married 64-year-old retired woman who enjoys a high level of affluence. She was originally from Connecticut, was raised Roman Catholic, and has a BS in Computer Science and an MBA in Management. DG retired several years ago from a successful career as a Project Manager for major corporations. She reported that she became disenchanted with the Church during her years at a Catholic High School and that her growing up years were marked by the toxic and emotionally abusive relationship between her parents. During her interview, she recounted how her disappointment with the Church during high school precipitated her moving away from the culture of her upbringing and that as a teenager she became aware that one of our purposes for being alive was to help others. This conviction was coupled with her adoption of an increasingly animistic worldview that resulted in her separation from the beliefs of the dominant culture affected by her growing awareness of her own identity.

DG said that she had been a lifelong seeker into the nature of consciousness and the linkage of all things through spiritual energy. She perceives consciousness on a model incorporating synchronicities, patterns, significant dreams, and the appearance of archetypal images. She claims to have a strong link to animals, especially the spirits of deceased pets, and the spirit guides she has encountered in dreams and journeys, as well as the existence of angels and extraterrestrials. Although she has never believed herself to be psychically gifted or creatively inclined, she expressed that she is now beginning to recognize some psychic and creative capabilities within herself. She believes magic to be a form of alternative energy that one reaches out to in a shamanic journey, and her increasing awareness of the sentience and presence of the sacred in all living things has caused her to gravitate toward Paganism. She repeatedly emphasized her sense of peace and power in the presence of nature. DG claimed that she believes in the existence of extraterrestrials and of people who can transcend time and space through their ability to use this alternative energy/magic.

She believes that she is only beginning her journey of self-discovery and exploration of consciousness and, therefore, lacks confidence in her abilities to heal, divine, or act as a psychopomp. She strongly believes in the presence of spirit guides and nature spirits and claims that she sees auras around living things. DG stated that at this point she was content in deepening her self-exploration and redefining her world through using techniques that she admitted were plainly alien to her as recently as 6 years ago. She said she followed her path of discovery intuitively through her Irish heritage and her strong affinity to nature. The images that she encounters during her journeys underscore her growing perception of oneness with the natural world, and the expansion of her perceptual boundaries, and that her Neo-shamanic practice seemed to her to be a greater step into the unknown.

The answers she provided on the questionnaires indicated a strong sense of mysticism, the efficacy of shamanic practice, and a strong belief in magic despite a professed dearth of anomalous experiences. She strongly acknowledged the presence of spirits, particularly nature spirits, and spirit guides. Although she reported that she frequently sees auras around living things, she admits that she does not perceive an ongoing communication with non-material entities other than a strong native intuition.

The answers that DG provided on the Mysticism Questionnaire indicated a strong animistic orientation, a sense of the multiphasic aspect of immanent divinity, and the presence of the sacred in all things. This represents a newfound sense of the veracity of the unseen which is significant for someone who has described her life as being deeply rooted and bounded by the rational and material paradigm of the dominant Western culture. Her answers on the Anomalous Experiences Questionnaire demonstrated a strong belief in the presence of entities unperceived by the physical senses despite a lack of direct experiences with such entities and phenomena. Her responses on the Magic Questionnaire expressed a strong belief in magic, but reflected her stated belief that she herself did not possess magical capabilities currently, although she made statements in the interview and responses on the Neo-shamanic Practice Questionnaire that she believed said practice to be a magical practice that connected her to the divine. She also indicated a highly developed sense of ethics and responsibility for anything that she undertook as part of her shamanic practice.

DG spoke repeatedly about her increasing connection to the natural world and said that she began every morning sitting on her screened in porch with a cup of tea and her cat while merging her own boundaries with the land, trees, birds, and animals passing by—a practice in striking contrast to the corporate world that dominated her life as an adult. Her reported perception of the images she encountered during her journeys and alluded to in her interview underscored her growing perception of oneness with the natural world, and the expansion of her perceptual boundaries and consciousness.

Participant 2 (SJ)

SJ is a 56-year-old divorced grandmother, who was working as a caregiver for the elderly. She was the oldest of five siblings in a blue-collar Roman Catholic household from the upper Midwest. According to SJ, the family was always very close, supportive, hardworking. She earned her Bachelor of Science degree in Speech and Hearing from the University of Iowa and upon graduation had professional success as a speech therapist and reading interventionist. She married an Iranian student and remained with him until their children were grown, after which they divorced. She says that she and her ex-husband remain very good friends.

SJ's interview was full of accounts of anomalous experiences and synchronistic occurrences, ranging from precognitive dreams to filming a UFO from her bedroom window. She explained that expanding her spirituality and helping others are the twin pillars of her existence and that these elements manifested very early in her life. SJ's interview and journey narratives reflected the dominance of her Catholic upbringing in her worldview. As a child, she loved reading about the saints and miracles and reported that her spirit guides include the Archangels Raphael and Michael, as well as the Virgin Mary, Jesus, St. Francis, St. Theresa and St. Rose of Lima, Peru. She stated that in her 20s she began to realize that hers was a spiritual path when she started noticing a marked increase in her intuition, sensitivity, empathy, precognitive occurrences, and prophetic dreams as well as an overall integration of the spiritual and material. She said that she views magic as an energetic force that is present in all of nature and the numinous and that she is increasingly aware of the presence of the sacred in all things both animate and inanimate. SJ said that to her anything that is miraculous is magical and has divine origins, thus representing the integration of the Catholic foundations of her worldview with elements of the shamanic worldview she more recently adopted through her practice. As she expressed it:

> Consciousness is life. It's life force energy, but there are differing degrees of consciousness depending on how much a person is open to their subconscious, and the unconscious and the collective universe. I believe that everything is alive…It's got energy so it comes from the source.

SJ claimed a growing awareness of a continuous dialogue between the material world and the numinous and acknowledged that she believed that anomalous phenomena and entities were constantly around us, albeit usually imperceptible with our physical senses alone. She said that she does not think "there are any boundaries between time and space. It's just like the quantum physics – everything is going on at the same time." Regarding her own magical capabilities, she stated that "Anything that I have I don't believe it is of me. I think it comes through me, not of me. I think it's coming through somewhere else, and I'm just used as a vehicle."

She talked about feeling out of step with the dominant culture since grade school and that to her helping people was far more important than material things, money, and honors. She confessed to not revealing her thoughts and attitudes to many people as a means of self-protection. Throughout the interview, she referred to her Neo-shamanic practice as being core to her life experience, and that, increasingly for her the inner and outer worlds were in constant and smooth communication and integration.

SJ's answers on the questionnaires closely corroborated what she disclosed in the interview. Her answers on the Mysticism Questionnaire indicated a very high level of mystical belief, particularly an acute awareness of immanent divinity, and those on the Anomalous Experiences Questionnaire implied a strong sense of the presence of anomalous entities and a personal history of supernormal experiences. Her responses on the Magic Questionnaire indicated that she had a strong belief in magic and its potential to manifest change on the physical plane, but that she herself was not a magical adept. She answered the questions on the Neo-shamanic Practice Questionnaire in a way that revealed that she believed such a practice to be magical in nature, and that it had the power to heal, help us to gain wisdom, and that she strongly believed in the validity of her journey experiences.

The influence of Catholicism and the belief in saints, miracles, and the loving presence of God, Jesus, and the Virgin Mary were at the core of SJ's lifeworld. She spoke repeatedly about her lifelong fascination with saints and miracles during her interview along with her perception of her guiding spirits as angels and archangels whom she regularly invoked to assist her in healing and psychopomp work. She claimed that these entities were around her at all times and that she continuously listened for their voices in the silence. She perceived divinity as being simultaneously transcendent and immanent and emphasized her strong connection to nature. Her journey narratives demonstrated a high degree of successful integration with the shamanic emphasis on the natural world and the Christian mysticism rooted in her Catholic upbringing.

Participant 3 (GL)

GL's background differed slightly from that of most of the other participants in that she is from the rural South and did not attend college. She reported that her birth father was physically abusive to her mother (but not to her) and that her parents divorced when she was 7 years old. She and her mother relocated to a neighboring state and her mother remarried a couple of years later to a man who considered GL to be his own daughter. Upon graduation from high school, she attended cosmetology school, became a hairdresser, married at age 19, and had a daughter at 21. She has owned her own beauty salon for over 12 years and is a well-respected member of her local community. She has an excellent singing voice and is a soloist at the Methodist Church she attends.

GL recounted that she could remember things from the time she was 2 years old, and that ever since she was a toddler she was aware of the presence of unseen beings, who she always referred to as "ghosts." She began to experience episodes of clairvoyance and clairaudience as well as lucid dreams as she matured, and that she was aware that she was different from other people around her by the time she was 3 or 4. Regarding this perceived difference from others, she said:

> I think I've always known that, always kind of sensed that just because I always knew that there were things lurking in the dark… There were certain rituals. I just knew once I closed the closet door and said "Stay in there," that I was telling the thing to stay in there and that it wouldn't come out, and it wouldn't bother me in the night. And I felt comfortable with that, and I felt I had the power to tell it "No!"

She reported that this early ability to achieve results through her use of will power improved as she got older and that she has seen this manifested many times in her life. She claims to use her will consistently to direct energy in her shamanic work. She differentiated that this use of will to effect change on the material plane was not magic, rather her consciously directing energy through her will in order to attain a specific result. In her own words:

> I just think about it and put energy into it so that makes it happen. That's my will – my will to make it happen… Magic is something that happens, whether you want it to or not. But I feel like the shamanic stuff is things that we focus our mind and our attention to and therefore, good comes from it.

GL further explained that others might consider shamanic work to be magic because they don't understand it and cannot explain it. However, she said that, to her, "It's all energy and it just flows with us and through us and around us and because of us maybe."

GL (like SJ) frames her shamanic practice and interaction with the anomalous phenomena and entities she perceives in a manner that is consistent with her underlying Christian beliefs. She believes in the power of angels to intervene in the material world and in the power of Jesus Christ to protect and intervene for the benefit of herself and others. She recounted an experience that occurred when she was pregnant with her daughter and had been very ill following a gall bladder operation. She recalled waking up feeling "paralyzed." According to her interview account of the episode:

> I know I was on my back, and my arms felt like they were physically pinned down. But I could not move. I opened my eyes and there were two Indians standing over me. There was a younger Indian that had long black hair and was kind of standing behind the other Indian. The other Indian had red glowing eyes and big gray hair that was waving everywhere and he was holding me down. And I could feel my stomach expanding and it was big. I could feel that he was trying to take [my baby] from me. I know that's what he was doing. And I was saying "No!" but no words were coming out. And I finally thought to just say "Jesus help me!" and, in that instant, the Indian vanished – the both of them did – and my belly went back down. And I felt like, "Okay. I'm going to be okay." But I still remember it like it was yesterday, and I *know* it happened.

This anecdote has many commonalities with reports of sleep paralysis, which will be discussed in Chapter 6.

GL reported that although she believes in the God of the Bible, she believes that everything is sacred (particularly nature), and that "divinity is just a divine energy that we all have within us and that it's connected to and through and about everything that we come in contact with in our lives." She said that she always senses the presence of her animal spirits around her at all times, as were the spirits she called "ghosts." She claimed to perceive spirit teachers only during her journeys.

This participant's answers on the questionnaires indicated a high level of mystical belief, a high occurrence of anomalous experiences, a strong belief in magic, and the frequent presence of elements of all three in her Neo-shamanic practice. Her answers about Mysticism indicated an enduring belief in the power and presence of divinity in her life, while her responses to questions about anomalous experiences implied a vigorous history of experience with anomalous entities and phenomena. Her answers to the questions on the Magic Questionnaire revealed a powerful belief in the existence of magic as well as a willingness to use her will to invoke and achieve results of healing, wisdom, or protection. GL's responses to the questions on the Neo-shamanic Practice Questionnaire indicated a steadfast belief in the efficacy of Neo-shamanic practice to affect healing, protection, and achieving powerful insights through journeys.

Based on statements and anecdotes revealed during her interview, GL has always been extremely sensitive to perceiving anomalous phenomena and having supernormal experiences, which she viewed as glimpses into a world that exists just beyond the scope of the physical senses. She was attuned to both nature and her ancestry (Scots-Irish) and has a particularly strong association with the spirit of her deceased maternal grandmother. She regularly attends Church but claims that she does not follow the limitations of Church dogma. She emphasized that she had a steadfast belief in God and the role of Jesus as a personal savior dwelling within all of us. Of all of the participants, GL was the most confident of her place in the world and the power of her own will in both the material and the spiritual realms. She believed that magic was an ineffable force that was expressed as energy that could be called upon in time of need, that good and evil are choices that we make, and that she existed in this time and place to help her family and community.

Participant 4 (AN)

AN was a 61-year-old mother of three grown children who was the owner, director, and primary teacher at a yoga studio. She has been a devoted student of Iyengar yoga for over 30 years and had the good fortune to be allowed to study with Iyengar for a month at his ashram in India in 2015. Yoga is the center of her worldview, as are her mixture of Buddhist and Hindu beliefs. Her family is the central focus of her life.

AN came from an affluent family due to her father's position in a large corporation, and she spent the first 11 years of her life in Rio de Janeiro and Barbados. She attended an exclusive British school for the children of diplomats in Rio and graduated from Princeton University with a degree in English. She was one of four sisters and said that the relationship between her parents was strained. She talked about how she found her father's presence to be forbidding and toxic and described how her entire world came crashing down the night that her sister was killed in a car accident. AN viewed the night of her sister's death as a turning point for the family and perceived that event to be pivotal in the final disintegration of whatever was left of her parents' marriage. For her, she said, the trauma of that night was pivotal because it opened her eyes to the reality of human suffering and burst the bubble of invulnerability, privilege, and wealth in which she had grown up. She credits the aftermath of her sister's death with her decision to marry her tennis coach—a marriage that ensured that her life was to be entirely different from that of the rest of her family. She said that she actively rebelled against the materialism of her parents' life, which she perceived to be a false and meaningless existence, and that she has never flagged in her ongoing rebellion against her family's worldview. Part of that rebellion has been her incorporation of elements of Buddhism in her philosophy and daily life, most predominantly her belief that all being is One Being, that all life is a sacred part of that oneness, and that the material world is illusory. On the physical plane, she believes that her children, yoga, and nature—particularly animals—have been her source of spirituality and comfort and have afforded her a sense of her own being as an integral part of Creation.

Despite the materialist environment in which she was raised, AN said that she loved to read and had access to fairy tales, which she loved. She reported that one of the most enjoyable experiences she had as a mother was to open up the worlds of magic and fantasy to her own children. She said that she strongly believed in magic as a child and loved that magic happened so frequently in fairy tales. However, she said that she compartmentalized the magic and the fairy stories and kept them separate from her everyday life, which was focused on school and sports. Her material world and her focus upon it caused "blinders" to be erected in a manner which caused her to cut herself off from the magic and stories she so loved. Her association with her future husband changed all that because he introduced her to the works of J. R. R. Tolkien, Ursula K. La Guinn, and other pieces of adult fantasy and science fiction. She described this as being a huge shift for her, because her exploration of these imaginative literary genres coincided with her sister's sudden death, the subsequent disintegration of her parents' marriage, and her mother's increasing inability to cope with the outside world.

AN regretted that her current perception is restricted by ordinary consciousness when she is not journeying. She said that she did not believe that she had any clairvoyant abilities, and that while she can frequently perceived the sentience possessed by animals and plants, she has never been able to perceive anomalous phenomena. She said that she thought that it was possible for her to transverse areas of consciousness in order to enable her to perceive anomalous phenomena outside of the journey state, and that she thought that

> Consciousness does put up the boundaries and the limitations but also has the capacity to cut through them – *Siddhas* in Sanskrit. I think it has the ability to focus on something very very small, but also opening up and being vast.

AN particularly resonated with La Guinn's concepts "about things being very small simultaneously with being very large," and the spectrum of time into past, present, and future, and connecting to some physics concepts was very liberating.

She spoke frankly when she acknowledged the dichotomy in her own worldview where, on the one hand, she recognized the presence and existence of unseen entities and magic, while on the other hand, professed her inability to perceive the non-material world at will. She attempted to clarify her thoughts on this puzzling matter:

> I get advice, but it doesn't seem to be coming from some sort of embodied by unseen presence. So, maybe disembodied, but I would give those things names, like maybe devas or angels, or maybe just pure life rather than coming from a being that I'm kind of jealous that other people see but I can't.

She expressed that this perplexity influenced her Neo-shamanic practice. "It depends on the definition of magic." She explained:

> I don't think of magic as a limited thing where you wave your wand and something happens. It's more like things that can happen that aren't explainable – like maybe rationally explainable. But then shamanism, it seems unexplainable, but it also seems to make perfect sense to journey to find aspects of myself that are available for guidance.

Conversely, she stated at several points in the interview that she had received guidance from the spirits of plants, animals, and rocks on her property, and framed these as being devas rather than the emanations of the spirit of the natural entities. In this manner, what she was reporting was that she was having experiences through the utilization of shamanic technology, but was translating those experiences to conform to her adopted Buddhist/Hindu model of making sense of the world.

AN expressed her strong connection to the Earth and the natural world in her interview and journeys. She talked about spending as much time as possible outdoors communicating with the plants, animals, rocks, the creek, boulders, and the mountain. She has given names to specific plants and rocks, much as one would name a horse or cat. To AN all living things are both sentient and sacred, and she treats them with reverence. She described herself as being a part of the Earth and nature rather than separate from them and reportedly lives her life consistently with that worldview.

AN's answers on the Mysticism Questionnaire revealed strong agreement with the statements implying awareness of greater consciousness beyond the sensate world. Her answers on the Anomalous Phenomena questionnaire reflected her belief in the existence and veracity of anomalous phenomena, but also her own lack of personal experiences with the unseen world. Although AN did not view herself as a magical entity, her answers on the Magic Questionnaire indicated that she believed in magic and had used physical tools such as ritual to focus her intent and bring about positive results. Her answers on the Neo-shamanic Practice Questionnaire indicated that she believed Neo-shamanic practice to be magical in nature, but that she herself was not the primary agent of any healing or change through her practice; rather, these were the results of the spirit world and healing energies moving through her.

Of all of the participants in the study, AN reported the most personalized relationship with nature and the world of spirits and also indicated the most permeable boundaries between her own perceived self and that which exists outside of her even on the physical plane. In these aspects, she would appear to have a worldview far more in common with that of traditional shamans than some other shamanic practitioners. Her journey narratives described Hieronymus Bosch landscapes which varied from the journeyscapes reported by the other participants in the study.

Participant 5 (GT)

GT was a married 59-year old who was developing an extensive organic farm and farmers' market and who stated repeatedly that serving the Earth is the purpose of her life. She endured a difficult childhood, which included physical and emotional abuse from her father, ostracism by the nuns at the Catholic school she attended as a result of her parents' divorce, privation as the oldest child in a single-parent home, and having what she called a near-death experience during a serious illness. Nonetheless she described her childhood as "good." She received a BA degree in marketing and later joined the Air Force where she served as a pilot. She admitted to being very rationally oriented by nature and that she did not open her mind to her own creative and intuitive aspects until she suffered a mysterious and debilitating illness. She possesses an encyclopedic knowledge of farming techniques and livestock husbandry, crops, nutrition, and herbal remedies. She said repeatedly throughout her interview that her garden/farm was everything to her and that if she cannot work with the Earth, she had no reason for living.

Unlike some of the other participants, GT recounted multiple instances of anomalous experiences. One of her earliest encounters occurred when she was about 6 years old and was sleeping in the windowsill of her parents' home in Shreveport, Louisiana. She awoke to perceive "a man talking to me through the screen." She roused her parents who investigated and found nothing—not even footprints which would have been observable due to the wet ground. She said that the man felt dark, old, and decrepit and that he stood in a shadow. Immediately sensing danger, she tried to scream, but that her voice would not work. She described it as:

> …one of those nefarious events that I can't say happened or if I dreamed it. But it was so real. It's still traumatic to this day because he was right in my face talking to me. And you wake up and there's this energy that is totally – it felt nefarious. It felt evil, kind of.

The incident she described as her near-death experience occurred when she was 12 and had been hospitalized for a high fever and delirium. She said that she had developed a "humongous" fungus on her face, and her mother (who was working at three different jobs to feed the family) had left her at home to rest, apparently unaware of the seriousness of GT's condition. GT reported that once her mother got home she took her to the emergency room, where she was given a scratch test for penicillin allergy. GT said that "I was so weak that I went unconscious, and the next thing I know, I was in the hospital in an oxygen tent and my mom was crying." She added:

> I sort of went out again, and I woke up in the middle of the night. And I don't know if this actually happened or not – it was a surreal experience – but this nurse came in and was messing with me. I don't even know what she was doing. But I looked up at her and I asked her, "Am I going to die?" And she never said a word. She kept doing what she was doing, and then she

melted out of the room and I went under gain. And the next thing I knew it was morning, and the light was… the sun came right in my window and it was like, "Oh! I'm back!"

GT also recounted a second serious illness that nearly killed her after she had been married to her husband, who had recently recovered from a bout with cancer. She talked about having chronic diarrhea for roughly 6 months, which left her weak and emaciated. She believed that it was this illness that led her onto the path of self-discovery. She said that she understood that she had to get well in order to work in her garden, and awareness of that work with the Earth was the "thread that kept me going." She realized that working with the Earth was her only reason for living. She said that she believed that this was a "spiritual illness that settled in my cells and I had to excrete it all…So that illness and recovery led me to yoga, it led me everywhere I am today." She reported that this was the turning point in her life, and the point at which she began to understand energy and sense a greater consciousness beyond the material world.

GT defined consciousness as "the amount of the cosmos that you are ready to allow into your viewfinder" and that she has been on a dedicated quest to expand her consciousness since her illness. She claims to perceive magic as anything that is fresh, new, and inexplicable and that to her "magic is the threshold of consciousness." She reported that this process is fundamental to her Neo-shamanic practice since it enables her to constantly stretch her limits of understanding, cognition and perception. To GT—and consistent with the traditional shamanic worldview—nature is very powerful magic that holds the answers to just about everything. Similarly to AN, GT applied principals of quantum physics to her experience of consciousness since it was that discipline that originally helped her to understand "the matrix and energy." She added that for her a mirror is magic and that she has had numerous prophetic and psychic experiences simply by looking into her own eyes in the mirror, and described one such instance that related to 9/11.

Based on her being raised Roman Catholic, and her fascination with some New Age philosophies, it was not surprising that GT frames most of the phenomena she perceives during journeys (including animal spirits and teachers) as forms taken by angelic beings. She described them as "fields of energy, vibrations, higher vibrations, souls in groups and banded together for energy and purpose. And my group, they will appear to me if I need them as an animal. They speak through nature." Sometimes, she said, they appear to her as white light. She says that she believes that if they are not embodied, then they are extraterrestrial in origin. She sees that as consistent with her belief in the limitless, unbounded essence of time, space, and consciousness. She spoke repeatedly of having conversations with the wind, birds, rocks, trees, and animals and emphasized that her close connection with the Earth was her "contract for this life." She expressed her belief in the sacred nature of all things and that divinity is a force constantly creating the whole of the universe and beyond. In her worldview, divinity "doesn't have opinions or desires, but there's a successful way to engage the force; and apparently, this force has some parameters of the divine plane, so if you're within those parameters you're in the flow."

GT stated that she clearly perceived herself to be on a curve of evolution, and that the more progress she makes along this curve, the less she feels compelled to interact with the mundane matters that she sees obsessing people in our culture. She said that when she must interact with other people that she tended to be very circumspect as to what she says and limits the interaction as much as she can. She stated that nature is her refuge as "the unedited word of the divine. When I want to know what the divine mind has to say, I simply look at nature." She believes that she is increasing her spiritual awareness so that she can "serve this planet. This planet is my love. It's just like she is the reason I live, and so the impetus for me growing my spirituality has everything to do with my mission while I'm in this earthly body."

GT's answers on the four questionnaires reflected the worldview she described in detail during her interview and replicated during her journey narratives. Although raised Catholic, the only thing remaining of that religious framework is her belief in the angelic beings she encounters, frequently presenting as elements of nature. The answers on her questionnaires indicated a high level of mystical belief (including a belief in miracles), encounters with anomalous phenomena, and an open mind toward the ineffable vastness of consciousness and beyond, as well as a strong belief in the presence and efficacy of magic within the parameters of her own definition of it. The answers to the questions concerning Neo-shamanic practice indicated that she perceived the presence of magic in the practice of Neo-shamanism and that she understood the responsibility inherent in the use of such a universal force.

GT professed to be comfortable within her current lifeworld and explained that she perceived her life to be a continuous unfolding of her spirituality, which she sought to express in her material existence.

During the interview, she spoke at length about her studies of New Age philosophies and her pursuit of spiritual wisdom through New Age gurus and (particularly) channels. She said that although she read many books, she found many of the inspiration writings that inspired her online. In accordance with the New Age belief that everything occurs for a reason, she rationalized that her childhood, which was marked by physical deprivation and abuse, was "a good childhood" and that it has served to place her on her current path of becoming a conduit of advanced spirituality in the flesh. Her journey narratives were consistent with the worldview she described during her interview, as were her responses to the questionnaires in that they expressed strong belief in New Age mysticism and imagery, numerous anomalous experiences and integration of the inner and outer worlds, belief that magic was a process that existed but was only magic up to the point where she understood its mechanism in any given situation, and that her Neo-shamanic practice was a viable way of interacting with the world around her.

Participant 6 (ON)

At the time of our interview, ON was a 21-year-old college student in her senior year at a local university. She is a gifted pianist working toward a BFA in Music, who decided to simultaneously earn a Bachelor's in Social Work so that she could do some immediate good in the local community. She is the only participant who is native to the area of the study and has had the benefit of a stable two-parent home for all of her life. She is very perceptive to the presence of entities beyond normal sensory cognitive perception and has demonstrated clairvoyant and psychokinetic abilities since she was a small child. She plays piano for a local Methodist Church, but expressed serious questions about the core Christian concept of the trinity.

She described her childhood in the rural South as being very good. She attended a local Christian school through tenth grade, after which she chose to transfer to a public high school. She said she always loved to read, play music, and enjoy nature with her cousins who lived nearby. She knew all of the fairy tales as a child and claimed that *Hansel and Gretel* was her favorite of these. She was only 4 years old when she began to demonstrate some *psi* capabilities. She recalls charming the king cobra on display at a nearby aquarium and described how the snake had its hood flared as she and her parent approached its glass cage. She said she just looked calmly at the cobra, who responded by deflating its hood and came over to the glass to look back at her. As she began to move her finger around on the glass, the snake mirrored every move of her finger with its own body. ON said that incident was the first of many friendly encounters she had with snakes growing up, including an event during which a cottonmouth peacefully swam between her feet as she and her cousin played in a local creek as children.

ON went on to describe another incident that occurred when she was about 7 years old:

> There was one my mom told me about where she was in her bedroom and I was sleeping on the couch in the living room… I was dreaming that either she or I had knocked her iron off the ironing board. And she said when I moved my hand like in that motion, that there was this bottle of nail polish sitting on the table and I was nowhere near it. But when I moved my arm that bottle went flying across the room…I don't remember it because was dreaming when that happened, but she woke me up immediately and told me about it.

ON expressed gratitude that both of her parents encouraged her to tell them about any unusual experiences she might have, and they both accepted her accounts as truth. She said that although most of her encounters with anomalous phenomena were interesting and benign, she remembered one occurrence that she admitted frightens her still:

> My dad would get up and go to work at 4:30 in the mornings, and it was about this time, and I heard footsteps walking towards my room. I opened my eyes and there was just this tall, lanky black figure standing in the doorway. It didn't scare me, but I just thought "Oh, well it's my dad," and went back to sleep. Well, the next morning I woke up and my dad had not even left for work. He said he had never come in my room like he usually did, and that he hadn't done it that night. And so a few nights later I woke up in one of those panicky, scared for no reason kind of states, almost like I had a bad dream. My door was closed and all the lights were off, and I got up to grab the doorknob, and I very clearly heard something tell me "No!" I was 9, maybe 10 years old. But I remember it standing in my doorway and being as tall as the door frame and with very long arms.

ON said that she always sensed the presence of something watching her from the corner of her room while she slept. She reported that doors that were tightly shut would frequently open of their own accord, and that she frequently slept with the light on in her room while she was growing up. She said that these occurrences and experiences made her feel separate from her peers. As she got older, she said that she became aware of the presence of angels and guardian spirits in her life that had saved her from serious injury in automobile accidents. She reported that she lost a good deal of her childhood sensitivity to the spirit world once she became an adolescent, but that she still senses things around her all the time. She reported that she saw a UFO streaking across the sky as she stood in the parking lot of a local Wal-Mart one night, which she described as a "very odd green spinning glowing thing that just shot across the sky."

ON spoke candidly about her views of consciousness. She said that she used to think it was simply awareness of one's surroundings and being able to sense the intentions of others, but that she has begun to understand that consciousness is far more vast than simply waking perceptions and intuition. She believes that she will realize greater understanding of consciousness in time and spoke about how journeying has considerably helped her to expand her view of consciousness. She went on to discuss her strong connection to the Earth, plants, and animals, as well as her uncertainty about what magic is and whether or not she has any magical capabilities. "Magic," she said, "was not really something I've been able to tap into. I feel like I don't know how to control it exactly. I feel like I could do a lot more if I knew what I was doing. I feel like I could become a healer. I've always felt that I'm meant to be a kind of leader, a healer…." She spoke of her belief that divinity is within everything and that the sacred is present in the entire natural world.

This young woman's worldview reflected her Christian education despite her current questioning of the doctrine of the trinity. Her answers on the Mysticism Questionnaire indicated that she held some beliefs (such as the belief in the existence of nature spirits and fairies) which were anomalous to her Christian worldview, but most of her answers were consistent with a Christian model. Her answers to the questions set forth on the anomalous experiences questionnaire reflected her history of personal interaction with unseen entities and anomalous phenomena. Although she answered that she strongly believed that magic is energy that exists to be used, she was consistently neutral in her answers to the questions on the Magic Questionnaire. Conversely, her answers to the questions on the Neo-shamanic Practice Questionnaire indicated a strong belief in the efficacy of Neo-shamanic practice for healing, gaining wisdom, and protection.

Benefits of Neo-shamanic Practice

In the process of writing this chapter, it occurred to me that it would be interesting to ask the participants and a couple other women in their spirituality and support group to re-evaluate their lifeworlds and their sense of well-being. Each of the participants had predictably encountered some changes in their lives since the original research was conducted over the summer of 2017. The "Neo-shamanic Practice and Wellbeing" Questionnaire consisted of 45 statements about identity and *Dasein*, well-being, expanded consciousness, and the integration of the mystic and the mundane and asked for the participants to list the three most important changes that Neo-shamanic practice has made in their lives. Respondents were instructed to judge the validity of the statements on a scale of 1 (strongly agree) to 5 (strongly disagree) with 3 being neither agree nor disagree. All of the participants in the original study and two additional practitioners received and completed the questionnaires in February 2019.

Significantly all of the participants had continued in their Neo-shamanic practice despite the pressures of some life altering changes 18 months after the original research. The great majority of answers indicated that these practitioners continued to experience the elevated sense of well-being, enhanced identity and *Dasein*, expanded consciousness, and integration of the mystic and the mundane evidenced in their initial interviews and questionnaire answers. The Questionnaire is included at the end of this chapter for reference. This would imply that the benefits of Neo-shamanic practice are (a) ongoing, (b) that the benefits are inter-related, and (c) that Neo-shamanic practice is a core element in the *Dasein* and lifeworlds of the people in the study. One has to wonder if the 100% continuation of practice rate and its positive benefits reflected in the responses to this Questionnaire would be seen in a larger pool of respondents, but that would be the subject of a future inquiry.

Elevated Sense of Well-Being

The questions in this section focused on areas such as creativity, everyday function, and connection to nature, and spirit. Four of the eight respondents reported that they had experienced an improvement in their physical health since they began their Neo-shamanic practice, and the remaining four was neutral. Six of the eight responded that they were experiencing a higher and more consistent level of creativity in their daily lives. They wrote about feeling more focused, attuned to their own needs, experiencing a more positive outlook, seeing more and better possibilities, taking things less seriously, and detaching their own outcomes from those of others.

Enhanced Identity and Dasein

The responses of the participants reflected their incorporation of a self-awareness and manner of being in the world that was based on authenticity, connection to nature and spirit, empathy, and improved intuition. It would appear from the answers these women provided that their Neo-shamanic practice had helped them to individuate, become comfortable in their own skins, accepting of who they were beyond the parameters of the culture and ego, and were solid in their sense of self and being. One respondent wrote that she felt as though she had a better understanding of her purpose for being alive at this time, while a couple of the others indicated that recognizing the healing abilities they possessed helped them to see themselves in a more positive light. As was the case with the other areas addressed by the Neo-shamanic Practice and Well-being Questionnaire well over 50% of the participants indicated that their practice had improved their self-awareness, facilitated the adoption of a positive sense of self, and enhanced the manner in which they interacted with the world around them and their place in it. The latter was demonstrated by a noted increased acuity in empathy and respect for their own authority and agency when dealing with the outside world.

Expanded Consciousness

The strongest common denominator among the participants in this area reportedly resulted from an enriched connection to nature. They wrote specifically about being "profoundly and intimately connected to nature," "being more in love with nature in all its forms and beauties," and "understanding the voice, vibration and needs of nature." They emphasized their heightened awareness of the wisdom to be found in observing the cycles and phenomena of nature, as well as turning to nature for the answers to questions. One of the participants stated in her interview that she perceived nature to be the voice of divinity and that she looked to nature to show her the answers to any questions that she might have. To these women, oneness with nature was a connection to the sacred because all that was sacred either resided in or was reflected in nature.

Dreams also were mentioned as frequently sacred messages, and the participants spoke about how they remember more about their dreams and understand more about what they might mean than they previously had. Likewise, the ancestors and the spirit world spoke to these women through dreams according to what they reported. Some participants cited increased acuity of intuition and awareness of the spirit world that exists just beyond the edges of our physical senses, as well as a sense of that ineffable force called magic being at work in their healing efforts and everyday lives. For these women, one of the greatest benefits of their Neo-shamanic practice was adopting a worldview that expanded far beyond the narrow physical-sensory parameters of the material world, and recognizing that they too were multidimensional and part of the sacred, natural world.

Integration of Mystic and Mundane

Through their Neo-shamanic practice and accompanying expanded worldview, the participants unanimously recognized that the mundane world and the mystical realms were partners in the ongoing dance of life. This conversation between the physical and the non-physical worlds was a part of 24-hour consciousness for the participants who made the following statements about the nature of its personal manifestations:

- "Understanding that everything has a purpose."
- "Accessing divine guidance for the benefit of others as well as myself."
- "Synchronicities."
- "Awareness of life beyond death."
- "Messages from other beings beyond the veil."

Seven of the eight participants answered on the Questionnaire that they had experienced an increase in what they identified as *psi* or anomalous experiences, including the perception of anomalous phenomena. (The eighth participants said she neither agreed nor disagreed about this.) The participants interpreted anomalous occurrences as part of their ongoing conversation with the sacred, which they claim to be within and around all that is. Five of the eight participants answered that they felt most connected to the sacred when they were doing healing work for others, and stated the belief that they were able to help others because of the relationship with the spirit world that is characteristic of shamanic practice historically and globally (Eliade, 1964; Ripinsky-Naxon, 1993).

	Believe	*Not believe*	*Neutral*
Elevated sense of well-being	101	4	14
Enhanced identity and *Dasein*	125	1	18
Expanded consciousness	139	7	14
Integration of mystic and mundane	131	5	15

Questionnaire had 45 questions in which elements of these four headings overlapped.

Used a Likert Scale with (1) strongly agree, (2) agree, (3) neither agree nor disagree, (4) disagree, and (5) strongly disagree.

Collapsed responses so that 51% and above answers of Strongly Agree and Agree were registered as Believe, 51% and above answers of Strongly Disagree and Disagree registered as Not Believe, and 50% registered as Neutral.

The responses to the 45 questions by the 8 respondents indicated that they all experienced an elevated sense of well-being, enhanced identity and *Dasein*, expanded consciousness, and integration of the mystic and the mundane worlds.

Conclusions

According to the interviews, Questionnaires, and follow-up statements of the participants both in the original 2017 study and subsequent review in 2019, revealed that they had benefitted from their practices of Neo-shamanism. They all reported that they had experienced an elevated sense of well-being, enhanced identity and *Dasein*, expanded consciousness, and integration of the mystic and the mundane worlds. They also reported that they had experienced physical and mental health benefits from their close connection with nature and spirit, and their identification as someone who could help others through healing. Perhaps the overarching benefit resulting from Neo-shamanic practice could be summarized in two words: Authenticity and Acceptance. According to the reports of the participants, each experienced recognition and acceptance of the authentic self. And belonging to a group that accepted the authentic self and re-enforced living in accordance with that true self encouraged individual self-acceptance and self-expression. This authentic self is Jung's individuated self—someone who lives in accordance with his or her internal being rather than someone whose identity is determined by the prescribed parameters of society's external dictates.

A great benefit of Neo-shamanic practice is its incorporation of the journey as a tool for expanding consciousness beyond the physical world, and perceiving normal, waking reality from an enhanced, multiphasic perspective. Such a worldview has the potential to provide a revised context for each individual to explore and integrate material consciousness with expanded conscious awareness, and reinforcing veracity of each person's meaningful interpretations of their own perceptions and experiences resulting in positive personal growth and self-actualization. The participants in the study claimed to have experienced increased physical and mental health, a sense of spiritual well-being characterized by a deep reconnection to the natural world, integration of spiritual and material realms, and an expanded awareness of the sacred present in all living things. They reported that they had developed an augmented sense of identity in relationship to all creation, increased empathy, and the realization that their lives had purpose and meaning. They spoke about having a personal relationship with many aspects of the natural and spiritual worlds, enhanced authority over their lives, and acceptance of their own agency to make meaning of events and phenomena while simultaneously analyzing the influence of cultural and personal lenses.

The participants professed that their Neo-shamanic practice provided them with a renewed sense of wonder, manic, and the workings of the ineffable in their lives, and they were thrilled to discover previously unrealized creative gifts and enhanced positive outlooks. The response of the participants in the study was the same or similar to responses recorded in the literature (Harner, 2014; McKinnon, 2012), and from other Neo-shamanic practitioners, the author has personally encountered through her years as a student, teacher, and practitioner.

McKinnon's work and the results of the author's 2017 study present the potential beneficial effects of Neo-shamanic practice on one's mental health and well-being through discovery of one's authentic self, consciousness expansion, modified *Dasein*, and integration of the mystic with the material aspects of consciousness. The next chapter offers a template for personal self-discovery which employs an integrated model including Neo-shamanic technique, expressive arts, personal mythology and dreamwork. I have used this model with great success in classes, but it is also appropriate as part of a therapeutic setting.

Appendix: Neo-shamanic Practice and Well-Being Questionnaire

Please answer the following questions on a scale of 1–5 as follows:

1 = Strongly Agree,
2 = Agree,
3 = Neither agree nor disagree,
4 = Disagree, and
5 = Strongly Disagree.

Please preface each statement with the phrase SINCE I HAVE BEGUN STUDYING AND/OR PRACTICING NEO-SHAMANISM I HAVE EXPERIENCED...

( ) A strong, profound connection to nature.
( ) An increased awareness and memory of my dreams.
( ) More vivid and lucid dreams.
( ) A sense of connection to the natural world.
( ) An awareness of the sentience in all living things.
( ) An ability to perceive messages from other living things and the elements.
( ) An enhanced sense of the sacred in all things.
( ) An awareness of my own divinity.
( ) Living more creatively in everyday life.
( ) Sensed the protection of the spirit world around me.
( ) Have perceived more anomalous phenomena.
( ) Incorporating journeying as part of my routine spiritual practice.
( ) Have noticed increased empathy with other people and living things.
( ) Have retained my ability to function in the material world.
( ) Have discovered an affinity with one or more of the fundamental elements.
( ) Have felt teachers and animal spirits around me.
( ) Have communicated with my ancestors.
( ) Have found that I have re-evaluated death.
( ) Have found that I have changed my perception of who I am.
( ) Have discovered a clearer sense of purpose in being here at this time.
( ) Have had glimpses of oneness and connection with other living things.
( ) Have ceased to make as strong a delineation between myself and "other."

( ) Have reassessed my identity.
( ) Have found myself interacting differently in the world.
( ) Been able to perform healing work for others at their request.
( ) Have noticed myself being kinder to others.
( ) Have experienced an increased sense of well-being.
( ) Have felt the divine present in all living things.
( ) Believe that other living things are sentient.
( ) Do not take things as personally as before I started my study/practice.
( ) Have modified many of my priorities.
( ) Have found myself less invested in the outcomes of particular situations.
( ) Have found myself living more authentically to who I truly am.
( ) Have perceived a shift in the world around me.
( ) Have experienced and observed synchronicities between the spirit world and the material world.
( ) Have found myself living more fully and more harmoniously with my inner sense of self.
( ) Have changed my perception of who I am.
( ) Have changed my sense of purpose and reason for being here.
( ) Have experienced an elevated sense of well-being.
( ) Have felt happier than before I started my study/practice.
( ) Have experienced improvements to my physical health.
( ) Have a rekindled sense of wonder.
( ) Have a heightened awareness of magic.
( ) Have an elevated sense of gratitude.
( ) Have a heightened appreciation of everyday things.

List the 3 most important changes this practice has made in your life:
1.
2.
3.

I give Dr. Karel James Bouse and the Institute of Esoteric Psychology to use the information provided by me in this questionnaire as a database for quantitative (statistical) analysis. I understand that my name will not be used, my anonymity will be maintained, and that this material is protected by the rules and ethics governing confidentiality prescribed by the US National Institutes of Health. I am over 18 years of age.

Date: ____________ Signature: ______________________________

References

Eliade, M. (1964). *Shamanism: Archaic techniques of ecstasy*. Princeton, NJ: Princeton University Press.
Harner, M. (2014). *Cave and cosmos*. Berkeley, CA: North Atlantic.
McKinnon, C. (2012). *Shamanism and spirituality in therapeutic practice*. London, UK: Singing Dragon.
Ripinsky-Naxon, M. (1993). *The nature of shamanism*. Albany, NY: SUNY Press.

CHAPTER 4

Neo-shamanism as a Tool for Self-Exploration

Abstract This chapter explores the benefits of using Neo-shamanic journey technology as part of a four-part educational curriculum for personal self-discovery. The journey is itself a deep meditative technique and has demonstrably worked well with expressive arts, personal mythology, and dreamwork applied to a model based on Jung's analytical psychology. Such a template has potential to facilitate a structured protocol to attain self-knowledge (*gnosis*) in a workshop setting, as well as an adjunct to traditional psychotherapeutic tools in a professional, clinical setting. This chapter presents and includes a detailed presentation of this Neo-shamanic-based curriculum.

Keywords Self-discovery · Neo-shamanism · Expressive arts · Personal mythology · Dreamwork · Jung's Analytical Psychology

> *You lack a foot to travel? Then journey into yourself – that leads to the transformation of dust into pure gold.* —Rumi

We have already examined the positive effects on general well-being reported by Neo-shamanic practitioners in Chapter 3. The shamanic worldview which is characterized by a strong connection to the natural world, a sense of the sacred in all things, and awareness of spirit and intrinsic,

K. J. Bouse, *Neo-shamanism and Mental Health*,
https://doi.org/10.1007/978-3-030-31911-3_4

immanent divinity, would appear to benefit practitioners through integration of mind, body, and spirit. Such integration has the potential to improve physical health, mental, and emotional balance and encourage a sense of oneness with both the numinous and the material worlds. An expanded worldview can offer the practitioners options for explanations of existential matters beyond those offered by the dominant cultural paradigm and its institutions.

It is possible for people who are not interested in becoming Neo-shamans to gain some of the wellness benefits of Neo-shamanic practice through using the journey technique as a means of deep self-exploration and discovery. The use of this technique can potentially open a new lens (or lenses) through which one's life and the world can be viewed, and encourage levels of connection to the world around us and depth to meaning-making not usually available through more mainstream cultural practices. This chapter will outline a curriculum through which this kind of self-discovery can take place.

Caveats

Before embarking on describing this course of exploration, it is important for the reader to understand that:

- Such a protocol is **not** a substitute for traditional psychotherapy with a licensed therapist.
- It is **not** a therapeutic regimen, but rather a wellness curriculum.
- Its intention is to facilitate expanded consciousness and integration of mind, body, and spirit. It is **not** a protocol for curing mental issues and/or personality disorders.
- It should only be approached under the supervision of a trained teacher or mental health professional.
- Deep psychological digging can frequently uncover repressed trigger points and traumas that can lead to emotional distress. In such cases, students should seek the help of a licensed professional.
- It is important to have a support system in place—friends, family, and other members of the course cohort—with whom one can discuss issues, revelations, and benefits as they arise.
- Participants are entering into an altered state of consciousness when undertaking journeys.

- Steady, repetitive drumming has been shown to trigger seizures in some people, particularly those with epilepsy. If you are one of these people, it is important to let the instructor know so that you are not subjected to the potential risks of the drumming, but can pursue the journeys through some other form of meditation.
- **Do not try this at home, particularly by yourself**.

Whither Self-Exploration?

Each and every one of us is a universe into his or herself, and the exploration of that unique universe is one of the most important and fulfilling things that we can do if we wish to live authentically and realize our potential. The technique of journeying that is used by Neo-shamanic practitioners is a useful tool for undertaking deep self-exploration because it facilitates deep, focused inquiry, and revelation without the risks and potential side-effects of drugs. Although there are definitely common denominators such as sharing of cultural influences, and common experience of historical events (such as the 9/11 attacks in the United States), the vast majority of the elements that constitute our own personal matrix are an individualized mélange of biology, family, ethnicity, transgenerational issues, personal history, and spiritual orientation.

Neo-shamanic technique is an effective device for self-exploration, particularly when it is part of a tool kit that includes expressive arts, dreamwork, and personal mythology. The directed focus of the journey technique along with the inherent cooperation of the limbic system with the cerebral cortex while in the journey state (Winkelman, 2010) allows someone to go deeply into specified areas of internal inquiry and discovery. Such a protocol can be used for facilitating personal growth and integration of mind, body, and spirit, particularly when applied in a framework based on Jungian principles of analytical psychology (Bouse, 2017). This curriculum is not a therapeutic protocol, nor was it designed to be an alternative healing device for people experiencing symptoms that require the assistance of a licensed mental health professional. It is an example of an interdisciplinary educational template that has proven to be effective for personal development and growth for the students that I have been privileged to work with over the years. Its goal is to allow the students to deconstruct the elements of biology (including genetics), personal history, culture, collective history, and learned spiritual orientation in a manner that facilitates their discovery of their own unique identities, and accept agency for their own methods of meaning-making. Family issues, trauma, transgenerational matters, the anima and animus, the shadow, death, wounding, and fear are all examined in journeys and expressed through expressive arts, and integrated with dreams, and personal mythology in a safe, confidential group environment under the supervision of a qualified teacher.

This is an overview of such a curriculum as an example of a potential application of Neo-shamanic practice for personal growth and well-being. Again, this is not a self-help protocol, and no one should take it upon themselves to undertake it without the supervision of a qualified teacher and ideally as part of a group. However, it is a system that if properly followed under the circumstances outlined above encourages the student to confront one's psychological issues as part of the housecleaning which is essential for the healthy discovery and integration of all aspects of Neo-shamanic practice, and the avoidance of the ill effects of spiritual bypassing (Masters, 2010). This work requires that the student be committed to the goal of enhanced self-discovery and amenable to acceptance of the potential changes that might occur as a result of it. Not everyone is all goodness, sweetness, and light, and people tend to butt up against some aspects of themselves that are less than heroic. All of us are examples of the Yin and Yang principle wherein there is darkness within the light, light within the darkness, and neither can exist without the other.

And from what I have observed through my experience is that students have a lot of fun throughout the process. Laughter may be the best medicine, but it is also a requisite for well-being and should be taken liberally on a daily basis.

Curriculum for Self-Exploration

The Jungian Framework

Carl Jung's template for analytical psychology provides an easily adaptable framework for self-exploration (Cambray & Carter, 2004; Shamdasani, 2003). The use of the four methods of accessing and expressing the unconscious described in this curriculum—journey work, creative expression, personal mythology, and dreamwork—is in keeping with Jung's contention that the unconscious itself was a valuable contributor to personal change

(Cambray & Carter, 2004). The unconscious sends its messages in frequently unrelated images unleashed within the context of a nonlinear narrative, and all four of the modalities of this self-exploration curriculum offer the opportunity for the unconscious to speak. Many of the images and phenomena that appear through use of these languages of the unconscious are similar to the archetypes of Jung (Jung, 1964; Smith, 2007). For example, the image of the wise old man named Philomen who appeared to Jung as a spirit teacher during his self-perceived mental breakdown into dementia, and which he documented in *The Red Book* (2009) in a series of stunning journal entries and illustrations is an image that many people report seeing in journeys. It is also an image that permeates our popular culture, e.g., Obi-Wan Kenobi of *Star Wars*, Gandalf of *The Lord of the Rings*, and Dumbledore of *Harry Potter.* And while it is not within the scope of this short book to examine the work of Jung, it is significant that his contributions provided the template for both psychoanalysis and the non-clinical curriculum we are discussing here.

Meaning-making is up to the individual, for they and they alone can string the pieces together in a way that makes some kind of sense for them within the context of their own lenses. Yet before the unconscious could be successfully accessed, it is necessary for those lenses to be identified and deconstructed. Jung's protégé Jolande Jacobi (1973) outlined the path of analysis of externals that need be assessed, identified, and evaluated before the rich reservoirs of the unconscious could be engaged. It is particularly necessary to deconstruct what Jung referred to as the persona—the identity interface we have between the external world and the internal worlds of the ego and the unconscious—before embarking on any deeper existential exercises. For many of us, the persona is an amalgam of externals that define who we are, what we perceive ourselves to be, and directly impacts our identity and *Dasein.*

The Persona

The Persona is a complex of external elements surrounding the ego, which according to Jung is the mediator between the external and the internal worlds (Jacobi, 1973). This complex represents the vast tapestry we have woven throughout the course of our lives to define to ourselves and the outside world and separate one from the other. The complex directs how we interact with the world around us and perceive ourselves. Therefore, it is necessary to pull the individual threads of this tapestry apart and put those threads in a new perspective in order for us to evaluate their value, embrace that which resonates strongly with us, and gently set the useless threads aside in order to make way for a new identity that originates from within rather than from external definitions. It is also important that we recognize the external factors that influence our lives and *Dasein* because they are what constitute our lenses, which are the primary components of our meaning-making apparatus. In Jung's schema, they are what stand between the mundane self and the individuated self (Bair, 2003; Jung, 1967). They regulate the way in which we see the world, and the way in which the world sees us, and how we interact with the world outside of ourselves.

Deconstructing the Persona

The **Mask** is how we define ourselves to the external world. The terms that are used are frequently societal identifiers reflecting our status and place within the culture. These terms reflect what we do, our level of education, achievements, accomplishments, socioeconomic status and represent a CV of our lives. The question "Who are you?" frequently generates identifiers such as mother/father, student, lawyer, son/daughter of ___, athlete, activist, Buddhist, animal lover, artist, etc. The next question is "What if all of that were taken away, who are you?" This question frequently generates silence because our personal identities are dependent on the labels that the outside world has selected to define us.

Once the external identifiers are removed, it is time to examine **Biology**. This is a fairly straightforward and nitty-gritty physical truth, but biology has a decided impact on how we appear to and interact with the outside world. It incorporates a mass of self-identifiers with all of the inferences both positive and negative attached to such things as gender, appearance, good or bad health, infirmity, age, gender identity, sexual preference, race, talents, and any number of other factors small and large that appear to define us on first glance. After biology, we examine **Personal History**, which is our autobiographies—the stories of our lives as we perceive them. This represents the narrative of what we have done and what has happened to us or affected us for good or ill since our birth. Investigating personal history gives us the opportunity to dissect and evaluate the influences on our lives that have impacted decisions we have made, fears we have embraced, what we have loved or hated, patterns that recur in our professions and relationships.

Next we leave the realm of our personal selves to examine the **Family**. Although we cannot choose the families we are born into, they nonetheless have a huge impact on how we perceive ourselves, how we make decisions about interactions with the world around us, how we perceive others, our core values, and our biases. A big part of adolescence is examination of family influences and the acceptance and rejection of some of them (Garrod, Smulyan, Powers, & Kilkenny, 2008; Santrock, 2009). A genogram is a useful tool to help people to map their immediate families through their grandparents, and even great-grandparents if possible. A genogram can note family issues such as divorce, alcoholism, addiction, adoption, premature death, and other potentially traumatic events and circumstances that can have a transgenerational impact on someone's life. It also can serve as a means of retrieving memories and family situations and stories that may have been forgotten but attain significance in recollection. These are all important parts of one's personal puzzle. **Ethnicity** is another factor that influences us in both genetic expression and transgenerational matters, particularly since current research is proving that traumatic memories pass from parents to child over generations (Furlong, 2014; Schwab, 2010). Ethnicity influences the family matrix as well as a transmitter of culture, collective history and traditions. A person who is of Latin American descent will have a different cultural history and identity than does someone of Japanese descent. There is much information about personal identity and *Dasein* embedded in ethnicity (Kremer & Jackson-Paton, 2014).

Culture and shared history are two other elements that are fundamental to how we identify and interact in the world. Regardless of our personal histories, families, and ethnicities, we are all living under the arc of the dominant culture of the contemporary West. The characteristics of this culture are materialism, rationalism, capitalism, and science. In this cultural matrix, veracity is given to things that can be apprehended and known through the physical senses. The positivist paradigm of science emphasizes the reality only of things that can be observed, measured, and predicted, and the spurious nature of anything that does not meet that set of criteria.

The high level of technology that we enjoy in our daily lives acts as an instantaneous vector of everything that constitutes the world we live in from news events, to music, art, film, and literature. People from the Baby Boomers through subsequent generations have lived with mass media in the form of radio, newspapers and magazines, television, recordings, and films as integral parts of their existence. Today's technologized media brings historical events, people, rhetoric, and values to us immediately in a manner that is both stunning and surreptitious in its instantaneous inclusivity through the Internet and social media. Members of any given generation are bonded by their collective experience through the media of major events and partially defined by that passive mass mediated participation (Becker, 1973). We all lived through the collective trauma of the 9-11 attacks, but only Baby Boomers are old enough to recall where they were when JFK was assassinated or when NASA astronauts first landed on the moon. We experience such events collectively and frequently emotionally through the media and thus we become simultaneously witnesses and participants. The events become part of our personal history and worldview because we were passively a part of them and likely experienced an emotional response to them. Popular culture likewise has collective cultural impact for films, music, and television are strong transmitters of taste, values, and morals of the dominant culture through sounds and images. These media generated and transmitted images potentially encapsulate semiotic messages that inform us and re-enforce the mores and attitudes of the tribe. As such, they frequently evoke a desire to conform to the tribal worldview in audiences; this is a throwback to our most primitive survival instincts (McClenon, 1997). They contain strong semiotic suggestions of how we should live our lives in a way that can ensure success and happiness within the framework of the dominant societal paradigm.

Finally, one's **Spiritual orientation** influences the way in which we define ourselves, and view and interact with others on both a mythic and a mundane scale. Spirituality is the manner in which the individual connects with the ineffable, the numinous, and the Divine. Initially, it is usually the family that provides the spiritual model, and in our current culture, the Judeo-Christian worldview has had hegemony for hundreds of years (York, 2002) having been spread through conquest, and conversion of conquered peoples or those in diaspora. Since World War II and the advent of the counterculture alternative spiritual orientations including atheism, agnosticism, paganism, Eastern religions, tribal religions from North and South America, and Africa, and the New Age have gained many followers as traditional organized religion has been in decline. Spirituality can be the bedrock of community and organization of one's worldview (Hood, Hill, & Spilka, 2009; Nelson, 2009), or it can be an invitation for someone to discover their personal relationship with the divine. Spiritual orientation is something that can fluctuate during one's lifetime depending on life events, expanded consciousness, social need to belong, or the ability of any given spiritual path to provide existential nourishment at any given time.

Deconstructing the Ego

Historically, psychology has been focused on the ego (Leahey, 2013). The ego represents the "I" that is separate from the "other." It is the gatekeeper, the survival coach that filters the external world from the internal world, and where many of our lenses reside. It is the sense of "self" that most of us embrace. In Jung's view, the ego is not the totality of the self, for the true individuated self operates and exists within and way beyond the ego's range (Bair, 2003; Jacobi, 1973; Shamdasani, 2003). In the quest to discover and bring forth the true self, the ego requires a bit of deconstruction, and the four modalities of this curriculum are quite useful in that process.

Some of the areas of the ego that require examination once the persona has been reduced to its components and subsequently analyzed and evaluated with the help of our meaning-making apparatus are:

- The Anima or the female aspect,
- The Animus or the male aspect,
- The Shadow or the dark aspect,
- Fear and/or the wounded aspect, and
- The Ancestors and/or the transgenerational aspect.

These aspects are quite powerful in our determination of the choices, decisions, meaning-making, patterns, avoidances, and attractions in our lives. It is important to self-understanding that we recognize these aspects of the ego because in such self-comprehension we have a better idea of what makes us tick. Frequently these ego aspects appear to us as symbols that appear in journeys and dreams so that it is useful to have the tools we use in this curriculum (or similar devices) to allow us focused access to these aspects. Once separated and confronted we have the chance of adjusting our meaning-making and sense of self to incorporate a renewed awareness of these aspects and have the capability to discern if an impulse, aversion or desire is being generated from one or more of them. Once we begin the process of deconstructing ego aspects, our new awareness might have the chance to provide us with new clarity and discrimination, which can translate into a modified and more beneficial *Dasein*.

The Four Modalities

Neo-shamanic Technique

Use of the Neo-shamanic journey technique is one of the four modalities constituting this self-discovery curriculum. It enables the student to access deep information relevant to the question asked prior to embarking on the journey. While in the altered state that constitutes the journey, the student perceives and interacts with phenomena and imagery in a direct manner relevant to the question being asked. It is then up to the student to make meaning from the experiences, phenomena, and information provided by the spirit world when they return from the journey to a normal waking state.

Aspects of Neo-shamanism—particularly the use of the journey technique and the connection with the natural world that is intrinsic to the Neo-shamanic worldview—are pivotal to such a deeply personal endeavor because it enables students to:

- Gain specific information in response to specific questions.
- Recognize alternative personal worldviews.
- Segregate troublesome issues and flag destructive patterns of thought and/or behavior.
- Create an expanded matrix in which to process and re-evaluate one's concept of the Self.

Both traditional shamans and contemporary Neo-shamans use the technology of the journey in order to interface with the spirit world to facilitate healing, obtain information and insight, assist departing souls to their new home in spirit (psychopomp), and protect their communities. The journey itself is an altered state of consciousness which enables the journeyer to perceive phenomena ordinarily imperceptible during the normal waking state of consciousness (Rock & Krippner, 2007). The shamanic worldview frequently includes the belief that the world of the spirits surrounds us just beyond the reach of our physical senses. For Neo-shamans entering into the journey state from a state of normal waking consciousness usually entails the aid of drumming to alter the brain waves to a dreamlike Beta or Theta state coupled with mild sensory deprivation through use of blindfolds or a darkened room. The result is a deep, meditative state in which the journeyer travels in spirit to meet with animal spirits, spirit teachers, nature spirits, and divine entities (e.g., gods, goddesses, angels, extraterrestrials) in an altered landscape in order to accomplish the predetermined and articulated purpose of the journey. In cases where the purpose of the journey is to learn about oneself, the experience is very similar to the vision quest of traditional cultures minus the severe deprivations and risks that reportedly characterize the traditional experiences (Eliade, 1964; Winkelman, 2010).

The journey provides a method of exploration by which students can come to face to face with the anima, the animus, the shadow, ancestors, and the source(s) of fear or wounding with the potential benefit of gaining profound information. I have heard students exclaim "Oh my God! That was my grandmother's trauma, not mine! I never understood why I was afraid of water before!" or things to that effect on numerous occasions. Journeys can provide clarification and insight into the meaning of dreams, reveal the source of repetitive patterns in our lives, uncover the source of seemingly irrational fears, and demonstrate how roadblocks can be overcome, and negative feelings relieved and healed. It is up to the individual to make meaning of the journey's gifts from the matrix of their own worldview and its components. In this way, the shamanic technique of journeying becomes a deeply personal experience that not infrequently contains the seeds of healing. The beauty of the journey technique is that it illuminates the issues underlying the individual's question. The following is the transcript of a narrated journey from the 2017 study that presents a fine example of how a journey is likely to unfold:

> I'm traveling to the lower world to ask the question "How can I personally protect and improve the local environment?" So I'm walking down the trail to my oak tree, and start looking for my root hole entrance into the tunnel. I grab the torch and proceed down the path deep down into the soil of the Earth. I come into the center of the mountain in the tree area and there's a shower of crystal light that washes over me, cleanses me. And then I proceed up the hill to the entrance, the opposite exit and then I come out into the open past a large rock. I notice the forest, the trail. My wizard advisor is there and he's pointing to go to the lake, go to the water. So I proceed over to the water, the pond. And I'm looking at the surface. It's very deep, it's dark. It's hard to see how deep it is. I'm wondering where the wild animals are – the ducks and all the creatures would be and I don't see any. Great blue heron circles and lands on the opposite shore and he's walking towards me. I'm watching him looking for something to eat along the shallows. He's coming closer to me. And I energetically pose by question to him – what can I do to protect this local environment? He seems to reinforce my thoughts about the vegetation has to be restored. The great variety of trees, the great variety of

> water plants. The animals can't survive without their food. It's a very intricate web of life and we need someone who understands this web to help spread the word as to how we might help to bring it back so that all may have a place at the table, not just the humans. The water is angry. The well water is angry. It's not good to consume so we have to get the springs flowing with more trees. I see a beaver is slapping its tail as if to applaud and agree with the heron's assessment. And the ground and look at the forest surrounding the pond to see if there are any other sins that are information for me. There's a blue flower – it looks like a forget-me-not that seems to be trying to get my attention. Now the air seems to be filled with more birds. They seem to be flying into the trees where before it was silent. It's almost like a council of wild creatures coming to endorse the importance of the water because water is the thing that all life is based on. All life on this planet requires water. So I thank the heron, and I thank all of the creatures for showing up to advise me. They all begin to resume their normal activities and fade into the forest. I thank nature for allowing me to speak for her. Now I am returning to the rock where my wizard waits, and I thank him for his support – for being part of my team. I return inside the rock, down the slope back through the crystal shower. I grab the torch and head back up through the tunnel and exit through the bark of the tree. And I'm back on my path in my woodland.

An important part of the protocol is teaching people how to journey. Not all potential psychonauts have the same innate facility for journeying. While some may have clear visions, others may take awhile to get anything other than impressions of phenomena. In order to get the students acclimated to the sensation and process of journeying, I have found that taking them through a guided meditation during which they return to a place in nature that has strong, positive memories, and resonance for them to be a calming and effective way to begin journeywork. After that I proceed by introducing some drumming and then add a guided meditation to help the students find the entrance to the tunnel to the lower world, and then another (using a combination of drumming and guided meditation) to allow the students to find their way to the lower world and back again. This procedure is reminiscent of learning how to ride a bicycle with training wheels. Eventually the training wheels—in this case the guided meditation—are removed and the person is able to navigate and operate the bicycle on their own.

Usually the client or class is in a quiet, semi-darkened room. Everyone is lying down comfortably and has a handkerchief or scarf to put over their eyes to further block out any light. The teacher instructs them to take 3 deep breaths. Then he/she repeats the question three times so that the participants can set the question in their minds. The question is usually framed as something like "I am going to the (lower or upper) world to meet with my spirit teacher(s) and animal spirit(s) to help me find the source of my fear." The drumming begins and maintains a steady, ceaseless rhythm. During the drumming—in which the participants are in an altered state of consciousness—they go to a place in nature that has generated a strong resonance within them, and either enter a tunnel to get to the lower world or to a high place such as a mountaintop or tall tree to get to the upper world. Voyagers would be aware that once the question or purpose is framed and articulated that anything that occurs from that point in the journey is part of the answer to the question. Animal spirits and spirit guides listen to the question or stated purpose and then either speak or demonstrate the answer(s). Although these answers can sometimes be predictable, in the majority of cases that I have personally seen people come back with information that is unexpected, along with reports of phenomena that they had never before encountered. The drumming lasts for approximately seven minutes and then the instructor plays the pattern to alert the voyagers that the journey is coming to an end, after which he/she drums the rapid return beat for a minute or so. The lights are turned back on but at a low level. The class then takes about 5 minutes to write down their journey experience, and draw the images if they choose, after which there is an opportunity for people to share their journey experience with the group or with a partner or triad if the group is large.

The ability to focus the purpose of the journey specifically is one of its strongest benefits. As a result of the interaction between the limbic system and the cerebral cortex during the journey both the rational and the irrational functions of the brain are operative and in communication (Winkelman, 2004, 2010). This enables the voyager to ask a specific question (or state a specific purpose), observe an alternative landscape and observe and interact with phenomena imperceptible in the normal waking state in answer to their question, and make personal meaning from the raw data acquired during the journey upon returning to the usual waking state. The participant's question is what drives the journey; he/she can ask for clarification at any time and likewise can abort the journey and return to a normal waking state at any point. If desired, the neuroscience of the journey allows the voyager to narrate the journey into a tape recorder while it is taking place, which can be a useful tool if one is doing deep work, and wants to have total recall of the journey (Harner, 2005).

In truth, sometimes journeys do not work. I have known people who have journeyed effortlessly for some time and reach a point at which they simply cannot seem to "go anywhere." This can happen for any number of reasons, ranging from use of medications, stress, hormones, emotional upset, or compelling mental focus on issues such as work, school, relationships, family, or any number of life's involvements. Often such a dry spell ceases after the compelling issue is resolved, or the use of medication (even antibiotics) ceases. On other occasions, a person's ability to journey can be jump started through patient use of guided meditations. In some circumstances, an extended inability to journey might be symptomatic of an underlying repressed trauma or other psychological issues that someone does not want to address on some level. Such issues tend to crop up in repeated dreams, so they do emerge at some point regardless of someone's desire to avoid them (Cartwright, 2010).

Expressive Arts

The expressive arts are valuable tools for both accessing the unconscious and expressing its contents because they are (a) nonlinear, (b) non-objective, (c) based in feeling and intuition, and (d) have the potential to represent the non-physical aspects of our psychologies. The use of expressive arts as an avenue of psychotherapy has developed as a viable means of giving form to aspects of ourselves that lie outside of the purview of traditional language-based forms of expression. Music, for example, is a non-verbal expressive medium which has the ability to evoke neurological changes in the brain that generate intuitive and emotional responses within those who hear it (Jourdain, 2002; Sacks, 2007). Anyone who has heard Beethoven's *Kreutzer Sonata* or has seen Van Gogh's *Starry Night* can attest to the sense of emersion into a realm beyond the mundane such artworks evoke. And while not all of us have the skill to compose a symphony or paint a masterpiece, we all have the ability to make a drawing, sculpt something out of Play-Doh, participate in an improvisational dramatic piece, write a poem, do something wild and satisfying with finger paints, bang a drum, blow into a tin whistle or kazoo, or let our bodies move in a manner that is more expressive than we can usually imagine (Csikszentmihalyi, 1996; Richards, 2018). What Dr. Ruth Richards calls "everyday creativity" is an inherent part of being human. Recognizing our everyday creativity is an empowering epiphany for many people. There is something almost transformative that occurs when one realizes and accepts that they are living their everyday lives in a vibrant and creative way be it cooking, re-decorating a room, solving life's continuous little problems, to hosting a social event. Richards' book *Everyday Creativity and the Healthy Mind* (2018) is an exciting exploration of our everyday creativity and how important recognizing it and using it is to our self-esteem, growth, and sense of well-being. It was recognition of the potential healing force of creative self-expression that inspired Natalie Rogers to incorporate its use into the person-centered therapy pioneered by her father Carl Rogers. Expressive arts therapy is now a recognized therapeutic modality to the benefit of patients and therapists alike (Mellick, 2019).

In *The Red Book* (Jung, 2009), we can observe the power of expressive arts to illustrate the visions Jung experienced during his interactions with Philomen. Jung was a fair man with a pencil and watercolors, and he used the visual arts to illustrate the phenomena he encountered and the visions that Philomen showed him. A good number of these illustrations present us with an inner landscape that is more dreamlike than based on what we are accustomed to seeing in normal waking consciousness. I have observed this same quality in the artwork, music, movement, poetry, and drama produced by participants in classes I have taught and in expressive arts seminars and workshops I have attended through the years. Much of this is personally powerful and inspirational to others, and all of it represents things that are not easily described through words. Expressive arts constitute a profound language unto itself, and it is this ability to give material form and representation to phenomena and experiences beyond the mundane that make them useful in a self-exploration modality. Journeys and dreams are full of anomalous phenomena and images that simply cannot be expressed in common language.

There are five basic branches of the expressive arts, all of which enhance a self-exploration curriculum. These are visual art, music, movement, drama, and verbal arts (including poetry, storytelling, and playwriting). **Visual art** can be anything from finger painting to film and anything in between. One does not have to be a great artist—or even adept at drawing a straight line—in order to benefit from making an image that is meaningful to them on paper. Collage is a satisfying mode of creating expressive visual art because of its eclectic aspects which allows for strong textures, and the added bonus that it takes the burden of drawing off of someone who is convinced that they cannot draw a straight line or anything else. However, I have both observed in others and personally experienced a sense of exhalation and relief when paint and paper meet to describe something seen/experienced in a journey or dream. **Music** has the similar benefits for both personal and group expression. Virtuosity is not required in order to grab a simple school-type of instrument out of a box, add voices and make a sound painting. Voices have remarkable ranges and applications, and it is no mystery why vocals and percussion remain at the heart of musical expression in nearly all cultures globally. Some people have reported hearing music during journeys and in dreams and have been able to reproduce these tonal patterns and tunes in songs, chants, and instrumental excursions. Some cultures believe that every single person has a special spirit song (Harner, 1982; Hultkrantz, 1992), and the experience of giving voice to one's inner being can be a powerful and liberating experience. Creating an impromptu symphony of voices, percussion, and simple wind instruments can be beautiful, rich, and evocative of journey-like visions.

Movement is the embodiment of a feeling or experience and is an accepted means of storytelling in many cultures. Movement and dance give our bodies permission to express experiences without the use of words and show our deepest feelings to the outside world in a manner that can generate personal and collective catharsis. **Poetry** is a unique expressive arts form because it uses conventional language in unconventional ways to make a unique sound painting. In poetry words and the spaces between them can be used to create rhythms, and tones in much the same way that a musical composer uses notes. Free form poetry has no rules and allows someone who might be intimidated by their self-perceived lack of artistic "talent" in other modalities to create something deep and meaningful that evokes personal images and feelings for others in the group. Poetry has particular significance because its sounds and rhythms can be easily incorporated into music to which others can move and become the core of a play or ritual. **Storytelling** is something that we all do. Humans are born storytellers. We respond to stories and consciously or not consistently share stories in our daily discourse. Mythologies and religious texts frequently tell stories, for we respond to narratives. Stories teach us lessons of life, such as Aesop's fables, and we can connect emotionally with a story in a way that other forms of instructional communication cannot. History is told as a story, as is the daily news. Stories engage us totally, and they are no less compelling for their frequency in our lives. Finally, **Drama** is a reenacted narrative that brings a journey or a dream to life. Drama in which the internal world is made external and presented in performance was a core element in the Gestalt therapy model of Fritz Perls. Drama can incorporate all of the other expressive arts and as such has been at the center of healing and religious rituals in traditional and indigenous cultures (Hultkrantz, 1992;

Sala, 2014). The simple reenactment of a journey brings that experience out of the realm of imagination and into the realm of material reality, and thus enhances its meaning and power.

Through using expressive arts, participants add an important dimension to their self-exploration, while simultaneously discovering and reinforcing their own creativity and identity as a creative person. Acknowledgment of such creativity has the potential to change someone's self-perception from that of a non-creative person to someone who has the ability to not only make some form of art, but (most importantly) recognize their creative potential and apply it in all areas of their daily lives (Richards, 2018).

Dreamwork

Jung believed that the unconscious was the greater part of our totality, a reservoir of personal and collective wisdom, and the origination point of seemingly irrational messages and impulses which nonetheless had innate significance in our lives. He wrote about the "autonomy of the unconscious" (Jung, 1974, p. 73) and believed that the disjointed, nonlinear, and symbols perceived in dreams held a wealth of personal and transpersonal information. Jung argued that dreams had intrinsic value as sources of wisdom, warning, and enlightenment that reflected the attitudes of indigenous and ancient cultures that viewed dreams as messages from the divine (Winkelman, 2010). References to the importance of dreams as emanations of the divine appear in numerous world mythologies, including the Bible (Avalos, 2014; DeConick, 2016; Harrelson, 2003; Leuchter, 2015).

While there are many methods of working with dreams, all require that the dream content be recalled by the dreamer. There are a few things that one can do to improve one's capability to remember dreams:

- Repeat the phrase "I will have a significant dream tonight that I will remember upon waking" three or four times before falling asleep.
- If you wake up during a dream, stay in the same position as you recall the dream to yourself.
- Keep a pencil and paper or recording device by your bed so that you can note dream images upon waking.
- If all that you can remember from a dream is a feeling, or a color, or a sound write it down.
- Keep a dream journal.

- Write down the dream as completely as you possibly can based on your memories of it. As you write, you will likely find that more details of the dream come into your mind.

Once you begin to make a habit of remembering your dreams you can begin to deconstruct their components by separating images, words, sounds, and the feeling they evoked. It is always beneficial in dream analysis to recall if there was anything specific on your mind before you went to sleep such as a problem that needed solving, a tense relationship, and concern for a friend or loved one, what you read or watched before you went to bed, images or events you experienced during your waking hours that made an impact, or even music you listened to (Moustakas, 1994a). Seemingly mundane occurrences can create a conceptual matrix for the content of the dream and could therefore have an influence on its meaning.

Dreams and journeys both tend to be nonlinear and symbolic. It is up to the voyager or the dreamer to make meaning out of the dream content. Fortunately dreams and their interpretations are the subjects of much fine psychological research from the 1950s to the current time. There are many resources for dreamwork and resultant methods for the analysis of dream imagery. Whereas journeys are undertaken at will from a waking state and for a specifically designed and articulated purpose, dreams—even lucid dreams—have no such controls. They simply occur as we sleep and can seem nonsensical, prophetic, enlightening, or frightening. The purpose of the journey supplies the context of phenomenological interpretation a priori. Dreams have no such framework and seem to spontaneously generate, leaving the dreamer with the task of making relevant sense of the dream imagery and experience (Bogzaran & Deslauriers, 2012; Cartwright, 2010; Moustakas, 1994a, 1994b).

Dreams, journeys, expressive arts, and personal mythology work synergistically to facilitate greater awareness and understanding of what exists in the unconscious. Workshop participants I have worked with have frequently reported that journey images recur in dreams and vice versa. Dream theater, in which dreams are reenacted, is a powerful tool for bringing a dream from the realm of the ethereal onto the material plane. Working in a group to collaborate on the possible meaning of dream content can be useful, with the caveat that ultimately the only viable interpretation is that of the dreamer.

Personal Mythology

During the 1980s people in the United States were reminded of the importance of mythology in our lives through a series of broadcasts on the Public Broadcasting System (PBS). These broadcasts were a series of interviews hosted by journalist Bill Moyers and the American scholar of mythology Joseph Campbell entitled *The Power of Myth*. Campbell had devoted his life to the study and analysis of world mythologies and was best known as the author of *The Hero with a Thousand Faces* (1949) in which he outlined the "monomyth" of the hero's journey from the mundane to the mythic through a series of trials, challenges, and mind-expanding encounters. This monomyth is a metaphor for Jung's process of individuation and Maslow's self-actualization, both of which are journeys of self-exploration. Campbell's hero was the inspiration for Luke Skywalker in *Star Wars*; in fact, Campbell worked closely with George Lucas who wrote, produced, and directed the film. Campbell revealed in his interviews with Moyers that the so-called hero's journey was a model that each of us enacted during our lives.

Myths are narratives—stories to recount and explain cross-cultural themes of creation, death, divinity, love, war, birth, humanity, and nature told in culturally specific schema—that manifest in the lives of individuals. Mythologies frequently link macrocosms and microcosms that demonstrate the relationship and interaction between the human realm and the realm of the divine. Becoming aware of our narratives and learning how to change them—and as a result the way we live through changes in our identity and *Dasein*—are the basis of personal mythology. Psychologists Stanley Krippner and David Feinstein devised a course for people to accomplish and manifest this process and change in a book entitled *The Mythic Path* (2006) that used a series of guided meditations and exercises. According to Feinstein and Krippner, we all have an original myth that represented our authentic selves, but this myth got derailed at some point on the way toward maturity, at which point we created a narrative that more accurately reflected our way of being in the external world. Yet at some point, the hero (in this case the individual) comes to a crossroads where he/she must decide to remain in the old outgrown prevailing myth, or face the perils of the hero's journey to discover a new myth/life narrative in which growth might occur and a new identity and *Dasein* can emerge.

In this curriculum, we follow Feinstein and Krippner's model of steps:

- Original myth,
- Modified/prevailing myth,
- New prevailing myth, and
- Integrative protocol for bridging change from old to new prevailing myths.

This model of personal mythology works well with other modalities of this curriculum for purposes of deep exploration, creative expression, and integration. Neo-shamanic journey, expressive arts, and dreamwork enhance the study of personal mythology, while the personal mythology provides a framework for analysis and integration that enhances the context of the other modalities.

Conclusions

This chapter has provided an overview of a possible integrative curriculum for self-discovery. There are any number of possible variations, additions, and subtractions of such a curriculum and are dictated by the needs of the client or class, and the goals of the teacher or therapist. Each one of the four modalities—Neo-shamanic journey, expressive arts, dreamwork, and personal mythology—can be effective in any combination or singly depending on the needs of the student. The purpose of any curriculum/protocol of self-exploration is to allow the student or client to engage with their unconscious, memories, and the elements by which they tend to define themselves, evaluate those elements and replace those what are no longer useful or viable with identity constructs that are more in keeping with the authentic self.

However, there are pitfalls to any practice that involves identity reconstruction and enhanced awareness of the unconscious, and Neo-shamanism certainly is no exception to that caveat. In Chapter 5, we will explore some of the potential pitfalls inherent in Neo-shamanic practice, particularly in instances where there has been lack of preparation through a supervised course in self-exploration and alignment with the authentic self.

References

Avalos, H. (2014). Nebuchadnezzar's affliction: New Mesopotamian parallels for Daniel 4. *Journal of Biblical Literature, 133*(3), 497–507.

Bair, D. (2003). *Jung: A biography.* New York, NY: Back Bay Books.

Becker, E. (1973). *The denial of death.* New York, NY: Free Press Paperback.

Bogzaran, F., & Deslaurius, D. (2012). *Integral dreaming: A holistic approach to dreams.* Albany, NY: SUNY Press.

Bouse, K. (2017). *Neo-shamanism as a developmental, spiritual matrix for contemporary magical discovery and practice* (Doctoral dissertation). Available from ProQuest Dissertations and Theses database (No. 10742675).

Cambray, J., & Carter, L. (Eds.). (2004). *Analytical psychology: Contemporary perspectives in Jungian analysis.* New York, NY: Routledge.

Campbell, J. (1973). *The hero with a thousand faces.* Princeton, NJ: Princeton University Press.

Cartwright, R. (2010). *The twenty-four hour mind: The role of sleep and dreaming in our emotional lives.* New York, NY: Oxford University Press.

Csikszentmihalyi, M. (1996). *Creativity: The psychology of discovery and invention.* New York, NY: Harper Perennial.

DeConick, A. (2016). *The Gnostic new age: How a countercultural spirituality revolutionized religion from antiquity to today.* New York, NY: Columbia University Press.

Eliade, M. (1964). *Shamanism: Archaic techniques of ecstasy.* Princeton, NJ: Princeton University Press.

Feinstein, D., & Krippner, S. (2006). *The mythic path* (3rd ed.). Ashland, OR: Innersource.

Furlong, D. (2014). *Healing your ancestral patterns: How to access the past to heal the present.* Malvern, Worcestershire, UK: Atlanta Books.

Garrod, A., Smulyom, C., Powers, S., & Kilkenny, R. (2008). *Adolescent portraits: Identity, relationships, and challenges.* New York, NY: Hill Higher Education.

Harner, M. (1982). *The way of the shaman.* New York, NY: Bantam.

Harner, M. (2005). The history and work of the Foundation for Shamanic Studies. *Shamanism (25th Anniversary Issue), 18*(1–2). Available at http://www.shamanism.org/articles/article18.html.

Harrelson, W. (Ed.). (2003). *The new interpreter's study Bible: New revised standard version with the Apocrypha.* Nashville, TN: Abingdon Press.

Hood, R., Hill, P., & Spilka, B. (2009). *The psychology of religion: An empirical approach* (4th ed.). New York, NY: Guilford.

Hultkrantz, A. (1992). *Shamanic healing and ritual drama: Health and medicine in native North American religious traditions.* New York, NY: Crossroad.

Jacobi, J. (1973). *The psychology of C. G. Jung.* New Haven, CT: Yale University Press.

Jourdain, R. (2002). *Music, the brain, and ecstasy: How music captures our imagination.* New York, NY: Quill/Harper Collins.

Jung, C. (1964). *Man and his symbols.* New York, NY: Doubleday.
Jung, C. (1967). *Alchemical studies.* Princeton, NJ: Princeton University Press.
Jung, C. (1974). *Dreams.* Princeton, NJ: Princeton University Press.
Jung, C. (2009). *The red book: Liber novus.* New York, NY: W. W. Norton.
Kremer, J., & Jackson-Paton, R. (2014). *Ethno-autobiography.* Sebastopol, CA: ReVision.
Leahey, T. (2013). *A history of psychology: From antiquity to modernity.* Boston, MA: Pearson.
Leuchter, M. (2015). Jehoiakim and the scribes: A note on Jer 36, 23. *Zeitschrift Fur Die Alttestamenthliche Wissenschaft, 127*(2), 320–325.
Masters, A. (2010). *Spiritual bypassing: When spirituality disconnects us from what really matters.* Berkeley, CA: North Atlantic.
McClenon, J. (1997). Shamanic healing, human evolution and the origin of religion. *Journal for the Scientific Study of Religion, 36*(3), 345–354.
Mellick, J. (2019). Piercing the mundane: The role of creative expression in transpersonal psychology. *The Journal of Transpersonal Psychology, 50,* 144–159.
Moustakas, C. (1994a). *Existential psychotherapy and the interpretation of dreams.* Northvale, NJ: Jason Aronson.
Moustakas, C. (1994b). *Phenomenological research methods.* Thousand Oaks, CA: Sage.
Nelson, J. (2009). *Psychology, religion, and spirituality.* New York, NY: Springer.
Richards, R. (2018). *Everyday creativity and the healthy mind: Dynamic new paths for self and society.* London, UK: Palgrave Macmillan.
Rock, A., & Krippner, S. (2007). Shamanism and the confusion of consciousness with phenomenological content. *North American Journal of Psychology, 9*(3), 485–500.
Sacks, O. (2007). *Musicophilia: Tales of music and the brain.* New York, NY: Vintage Books.
Sala, L. (2014). *Ritual: A magical perspective.* New Delhi, IN: Nirala.
Santrock, J. (2009). *Life-span development.* New York, NY: McGraw-Hill Higher Education.
Schwab, J. (2010). *Haunting legacies: Violent histories and transgenerational trauma.* New York, NY: Columbia University Press.
Shamdasani, S. (2003). *Jung and the making of modern psychology: A dream of a science.* New York, NY: Cambridge University Press.
Smith, C. (2007). *Jung and shamanism in dialogue.* New York, NY: Paulist.
Winkelman, M. (2004). Shamanism as the original neurotheology. *Zygon, 39*(1), 193–217.
Winkelman, M. (2010). *Shamanism: A biopsychosocial paradigm of consciousness and healing* (2nd ed.). Santa Barbara, CA: Praeger.
York, M. (2002). *Pagan theology: Paganism as a world religion.* New York, NY: New York University Press.

CHAPTER 5

Potential Pitfalls of Neo-shamanic Practice

Abstract This chapter describes the pitfalls that can occur to those practicing Neo-shamanism and embracing its accompanying anomalous worldview. Neo-shamanic practice and its resultant awareness of the sacred aspects of the mundane world as well as the existence of a world beyond material consensual reality that is imperceptible with the physical senses tend to place practitioners in a state of chronic cultural dissonance. It is tempting for Neo-shamanic practitioners to turn to spiritual means of dealing with mundane and psychological issues and traumas rather than seeking more culturally sanctioned sources of assistance such as psychotherapy. This spiritual bypassing can result in a failure to adequately resolve the problems at hand. It can also lead to identity dysfunctions, including grandiosity, intensified fantasy proneness (which can present in conditions such as sleep paralysis), and intensified schizotypy. While elements of fantasy proneness and schizotypy can enhance creativity, they have the potential to develop into full-fledged psychological disorders and/or sociological dysfunction if not balanced by connection to the material world through relationships, professional assistance, or a well-grounded identity and integrated *Dasein*.

Keywords Cultural dissonance · Spiritual bypassing · Dysfunction identity · Grandiosity · Fantasy proneness · Sleep paralysis · Schizotypy

K. J. Bouse, *Neo-shamanism and Mental Health*,
https://doi.org/10.1007/978-3-030-31911-3_5

Whoever travels without a guide needs two hundred years for a two day journey.
—Rumi

We have established that Neo-shamanic technique can be a valuable tool for consciousness research and self-exploration and also that the practice of Neo-shamanism has the potential to act as a portal toward an expanded consciousness, sense of well-being, and a heightened experience of being in the world. In addition, Neo-shamanism is a spirituality-based technology that can provide a valuable means of mind-body-spirit integration in a therapeutic setting (McKinnon, 2012). However, like anything else, Neo-shamanic practice—particularly if undertaken without the necessary deconstructive exercise of self-exploration and without supervision and a supportive group environment—harbors intrinsic pitfalls. The most prevalent of these are the results of cultural dissonance, spiritual bypassing, and the development of dysfunctional identity issues that impair someone's capability of healthy interaction with the world around them. The latter might manifest as grandiosity, dissociative worldview, and anti-social behavior, as well as intensified fantasy proneness and schizotypy.

Neo-shamanism: Spiritual Technology or Psychopathology?

Neo-shamanism is the practice of traditional shamanic techniques by contemporary Western practitioners so that they might draw on expanded, non-ordinary consciousness to facilitate healing of others and obtain information from the spirit world in order to benefit other individuals and the community (Krippner, 2000). Although much of the literature represents the research of anthropologists (Eliade, 1964; Harner, 1982; McClenon, 1997; Walsh, 1992; Winkelman, 2004, 2010), contributions from psychologists (notably Rock and Krippner) began to appear around 2000. These psychological inquiries produced research that was based on a more scientific model than the ethnographic and artifact-based studies of the anthropologists (Rock & Krippner, 2008a, 2008b, 2008c).

The popularity of Harner's *The Way of the Shaman* (1982) and his workshops were partially responsible for the development of Neo-shamanism in the United States and Europe. Neo-shamanism emerged from the New Age movement of the 1980s and 1990s, and along with Neo-paganism and Wicca, represented the emergence of a subculture embracing a strong magical element that was anomalous to the materialistic worldview of Abrahamic faith-based dominant Western societies (Wallis, 2003). The similarity of phenomena experienced by members of this magical subculture was consistent with some symptoms of schizotypy accepted by the mental health establishment (American Psychiatric Association, 2013; Polimeni, 2012) and accentuated the inherent cultural dissonance between a magical worldview and a materialist cultural paradigm. The result of this perceptual dichotomy was the pathologizing of the anomalous belief system by the institutions of the overarching culture.

Winkelman (2004, 2009, 2010) made significant interdisciplinary contributions to the study of shamanism, drawing from the fields of neuroscience, anthropology, and religion. He argued that rather than being an anomalous schizotypal behavior as defined by our current culture, the shamanic *weltanschauung* (including its practices) was something that represented the earliest means by which humans interacted with the sacred for reasons of healing, survival, and wisdom (Winkelman, 2004, 2009). Winkelman's conclusions were reinforced by the findings of other researchers (McClenon, 2011; Rock, Abbott, Childargushi, & Kiehne, 2008). Rock and his colleagues explored and compared the phenomena perceived by highly cognitively perceptive participants who were exposed to shamanic drumming with participants who were sitting in meditation (Rock et al., 2008). They observed that the perceived phenomena of the participants influenced by the drumming were reportedly more vivid and culturally anomalous than that of the other participants (McClenon, 2011; Rock et al., 2008; Winkelman, 2004). Rock's research team reported in 2008 that the phenomena perceived by the participants under the influence of shamanic drumming were of a nature usually associated with schizotypy by Western clinical psychologists. However, the team made the determination that the reported phenomena were in fact not schizotypal because the participants demonstrated the ability to control their interactions with the perceived phenomena.

Kremer (2004) postulated that shamanic practice resonated with both contemporary and archaic practitioners because of the ability of the brain to integrate the mundane and personal with the mythic, archetypal, and transpersonal realms, which constitute the seat of religion. Other researchers in Europe performed similar research with shamanic drumming and determined that shamanic journeys promised to be a valuable adjunct to traditional psychotherapy protocols (Kjellgren & Erickson,

2013; McKinnon, 2012). Rock was particularly diligent in his exploration of shamanic experience and phenomena using accepted scientific models, protocols, and tests such as the Watkins Affect Bridge (Rock & Baynes, 2005) and the Phenomenology of Consciousness Inventory (Pekala, 1991). By subjecting shamanic experience and perceived phenomena to investigation on the scientific model, researchers such as Rock, Krippner, and Winkelman created a model of sensory-based phenomenological data that can be drawn upon by other researchers to strengthen the argument that cultural dissonance in the form of spiritual belief and practice is not synonymous with psychopathology.

Cultural Dissonance

Neo-shamanism is an alien practice in the contemporary Euro-centric societies and dominant cultures of Europe, North and South America, and Australia. These same areas are home to groups in diaspora from Africa, the Middle East, and Asia that migrated to the areas dominated by European culture through slavery, displacement, and pursuit of economic opportunities. Native groups continue to reside in the parts of the world colonized by Europeans. The foundation of our contemporary dominant culture in the colonized lands was imported from Europe initially through conquest followed by mass immigration and plantation of European settlers who reinforced that culture in their new homes. They replicated European institutions to uphold European values, religion, economics, and worldviews, which embraced materialism, monotheism, and science. Pockets of shamanic practices and worldviews continued to exist in communities of native peoples and immigrants from places like Africa, but they were frequently subject to persecution by the European majority in the name of progress. Many of today's Neo-shamanic practitioners are the descendents of those European colonists and were raised within the post-Reformation cultural paradigm of their European ancestors. Shamanic practice and beliefs lie far outside of that paradigm, which views such lifeways as primitive, ill-conceived, and potentially dangerous. This point of view is incorporated in the institutions of contemporary Western culture, including education, medicine, science, and psychology.

This situation represents a stressor for contemporary Western Neo-shamanic practitioners because they are dipping into waters that are uncharted. Some of their beliefs are so far outside of the parameters of the dominant cultural paradigm that those operating within those cultural boundaries frequently perceive shamanic practice and worldview as deviant and pathological. Neo-shamanic practitioners therefore might experience a sense of cultural dissonance and disapproval. The participants in the 2017 study unanimously spoke of the vigilance and discretion with which they lived their lives. Some of them claimed that they avoided mainstream society as much as possible withdrawing to their close friends and families. Others claimed to clothe themselves in a role or don a mask during any interactions with others outside of family and close friends. One participant admitted that she had been with her fiancé for three years before telling him about her unusual beliefs. Being at odds with the worldview and practices prevalent in one's society is always a risky business because the result can lead to isolation from the tribe and/or a negation of one's capability to function rationally (McClenon, 1997, 2011). Human beings are social animals who are dependent on society in large part for the meeting of basic survival needs, and isolation could have serious and even life-threatening consequences. The crux of this is that Neo-shamanism is a contemporary practice that is at odds with dominant societal attitudes. The combination of lack of societal support and risk of societal censure makes it difficult for some Neo-shamanic practitioners to live their lives in the world authentically, which has a negative impact on their *Dasein*.

Neo-shamanic practitioners seeking a supportive cultural matrix are frequently drawn to alternative spiritual communities. The New Age movement and Neo-paganism are two such spirituality-based subcultural groups that can provide welcome and community to Neo-shamanic practitioners.

Spiritual Bypassing

The late clinical psychologist John Welwood used the term "spiritual bypassing" in 1984 to describe the use of spiritual beliefs and practices as means of overriding and avoiding painful issues (Masters, 2010). According to Masters (2010), spiritual bypassing tends to occur when someone embraces a spirituality-based practice (such as Neo-shamanism) and uses it as a substitute for dealing with the traumas, repressed emotions, fears, and negative patterns that we all carry with us and which working with a skilled therapist can do much to integrate and alleviate. In other words, spiritual bypassers tend to use not only spiritual practice, but a fantasy-based identity derived from that practice, as a band-aid to cover unhealed psychological and emotional wounds. The New Age platitudes that "Everything happens for a reason" and "It's all for the good" can become rationalizations for those who desire to keep their personal pain at bay through avoidance rather than confronting it. Masters (2010) further cites magical thinking and over-permeable boundaries as characteristics of both New Age attitudes and spiritual bypassing.

Spiritual bypassing is recognized by psychologists as a coping mechanism used by some people to leave their negative experiences behind and create a new identity based on their spiritually derived conception of who they are. Its manifestation in beliefs and practices is expressed on a spectrum and is highly individualized. Fox, Cashwell, and Picciotto (2017) recognized that one of the difficulties in dealing with spiritual bypassing therapeutically was the lack of any tool to measure and screen the degree and particulars of the bypass mechanism. They developed the Spiritual Bypass Scale-13 (SBS-13) to analyze what they determined to be the two key elements present in spiritual bypassing, namely psychological avoidance and spiritualizing. The test is based on statements, e.g., "I believe it is preferable to cure emotional problems by being spiritually advanced" (2017, p. 277) to be answered Strongly Agree, Agree, Disagree, and Strongly Disagree which are then measured on a Likert scale. It was the hope of the researchers that the SBS-13 was an initial (albeit incomplete) tool to aid therapists in the recognition and treatment of spiritual bypassing.

The primary hazard with spiritual bypassing is that one's identity and accompanying self-esteem and *Dasein* has no solid foundation, so that when life throws a curveball (as it has been known to do) the bypasser's house of cards tumbles down about them. Masters (2010) likened this occurrence to someone living in the penthouse of a seven-story building with a rotten foundation and deteriorating walls, ceilings, trusses, and floors in between. Welwood (1979) accentuated the need for a stable "self-structure" (p. 65) and believed that people who were unsuccessful in their navigation of the developmental life path outlined by Erikson (1980) tended to use spirituality as a means of filling the gaps. Rather than process the psychological cause for their emotional pain, spiritual bypassers opt for the perceived spiritual high of self-perception above the pain level.

Likewise spiritual bypassing can be used as a means of avoiding the shadow aspects of the self. Clarke, Giordano, Cashwell, and Lewis (2013) observed from a counseling perspective that spiritual bypassers frequently exhibited "…the need to control others and the self, dichotomous thinking, shame, fear, emotional confusion, addiction, high tolerance for inappropriate behavior, codependence…" (p. 88). They argue that individuals who are engaging in spiritual practices to avoid confronting, examining, and resolving their psychological issues frequently discover that they cannot satisfactorily sustain their spirituality and imagined wellness since the underlying issues continue to erode their false sense of well-being from within. They recommend that counselors working with people in spiritual bypass need to recognize the bypass as a coping strategy and proceed in a person-centered, reflexive, and empathic manner to validate the anxiety, fear, and/or shame that the client might experience as a result of the underlying issues. Unfortunately, spiritual bypassers are more likely to seek advice from spiritual advisors or authority figures or turn to exaggerated spiritual practice rather than engaging the help of a therapist when the inevitable problems arise (2013, p. 89).

Spiritual bypassing poses a major pitfall for Neo-shamanic practitioners who by virtue of their practices and beliefs can exist in two separate realms of consciousness simultaneously. In order to navigate this perceptual dichotomy and remain integrated and functional, it is necessary that the individual practitioner establishes and maintains a clear sense of boundaries. Another driver cutting you off in traffic is not a spiritually significant occurrence or a magical sign of something else. It is a hazard at worst and an annoyance at best perpetrated by another human being who is either distracted, impaired, incompetent, or just rude. I make sure to tell my students repeatedly that there are plenty of times when a rock is simply a rock.

The pitfalls of spiritual bypassing underscore the importance for working through one's inner landscape with all of its crannies, caves, and monsters with a therapist or through a supervised teaching curriculum prior to undertaking the task of performing shamanic work of any kind for others. Unresolved psychological matters such as traumas, repressed emotions, fears, and gaps in the developmental process invariably come roaring up during the course of journeywork. Since much of the information acquired through journeywork is in the form of images, their meaning and significance are dependent upon the interpretative lenses of the practitioner underscoring the importance of each person knowing from a rational perspective what those lenses are. Lack of integration of rational and irrational processes, particularly where there is lack of community or group support, can lead to dependence upon magical thinking and/or the adoption of a magic-based persona that could result in impaired functionality in the normal waking state. Having a strong sense of grounded identity and purpose within the material world is essential to the mental health of Neo-shamanic practitioners, as is having a strong support group and access to a good therapist.

Practitioners who are engaged in spiritual bypassing should resist the urge to simply journey on an issue that arises, keeping in mind that the spiritual entities with whom they interact during journeys operate outside of space and time, and tend to be ambivalent and vague leaving the hapless practitioner at the mercy of their own interpretative lenses and subsequent landmine-riddled meaning-making processes.

Dysfunctional Identity

In essence, identity is the sense and definition of one's self. It is based on a convergence of biological, psychological and emotional, ethnic, cultural, and spiritual factors. It incorporates our core values, beliefs, creativity, and perception of the world around us as well as our dreams, boundaries, and interactions. Identity is what determines our self-esteem and ultimately influences our *Dasein*. Jung based his system of analytical psychology on the discovery and differentiation (individuation) of the core authentic self that is the basis of who we are, as opposed to the persona/mask or the self dictated by the outside world. The individuated self is who we know ourselves to be without the trappings and judgments of outside elements, and it is knowledge and internalization of this individuated self that enables us to live with a sense of purpose and enrich our lives with meaning and authenticity. Neo-shamanic practice can be a valuable piece of our total identity puzzle provided it is integrated and balanced with other aspects that may be somewhat less esoteric. Difficulties can arise when a Neo-shamanic practice—which is the use of a spirit-based, esoteric, ancient, irrational technology to assist others with problems in a rational, material, positivist society—is not fully integrated by the practitioner into the totality of the individual. As exciting and fulfilling as it may be to use Neo-shamanism to interface with the world beyond material, sensate boundaries for the benefit of others through healing and insight, it must be balanced with the willingness and ability to do the grocery shopping, go to work, have successful relationships, and balance the checkbook. When this balance is lost due to incomplete integration, it is important that the practitioner steps back and recognizes that there is likely some additional psychological work to be done.

Like it or not, we all must function within the parameters of our contemporary Western culture. "Neo-shamanic practitioner" is not a job title according to the US Department of Labor, nor is it an appropriate answer under "Occupation" when filling out one's annual income tax returns or applying for a passport. Neo-shamanic practitioners frequently inhabit life-worlds and have core values that are not reflected in the dominant culture of the contemporary West. How to navigate that cultural dissonance and to live simultaneously functionally and authentically is a challenge facing some practitioners. Each must find his or her own balance point, keep firm boundaries, nourish and exercise a healthy sense of humor (particularly where oneself is concerned), and appreciate the ongoing dance between the material world and the world of spirits and anomalous phenomena. Loss of that balance contains the risk of the development of a dysfunctional identity which might manifest in ways that are interpreted to be evidence of disorders by contemporary psychological practice. The most likely of these are grandiosity, intensified fantasy proneness, and intensified schizotypal behavior. None of these behaviors are functionally debilitating in and of themselves. To the contrary, particularly fantasy proneness and schizotypal tendencies have been linked to creativity (Richards, 2001, 2009; Richards & Kinney, 1990). Yet if left unchecked, they have the potential to undermine the ability of an individual to successfully function and enjoy life or, in the most extreme cases, evolve into a full-fledged disorder. According to evolutionary psychology, the same gene responsible for the ability to journey and interact with the supernormal world is also responsible for schizophrenia (Armstrong, 2010; Stevens & Price, 2006).

Grandiosity

Grandiosity is the belief that one is greater and more important than they actually are (VandenBos, 2015). According to *DSM-V* (2013), grandiosity (a/k/a inflated self-belief) can be symptomatic of narcissism and schizotypy. Someone in the thrall of grandiose self-delusion treads close to the line of anti-social behavior as the perceived separation between the Self and Others widens. Because the Neo-shamanic practitioner operates within the mythic and supernormal realms during journeys, there is the risk that they might carry over their journey aspect into normal, waking consciousness in the material world. The world of journeywork can encourage a poorly grounded practitioner who wishes to override traumas and disappointments to become what they want to be. The journey can offer a playing field to one's inner Walter Mitty (Thurber, 2016). If a Neo-shaman removes an illness-causing spirit intrusion from a client suffering from the flu, it is essential that they settle back into their identity in the mundane world once the healing journey is completed. Eating something, talking to a friend or family member, listening to some good music, watching a favorite movie, or even doing the laundry can assist in a practitioner's successful re-entry into contemporary twenty-first-century life. It is frequently the solitary practitioner who over-identifies with the otherworldly aspects of Neo-shamanic practice, is lacking social and/or professional support, and who has permeable or insufficient boundaries who is most at risk for adopting a grandiose persona.

Intensified Fantasy Proneness and Incidents of Sleep Paralysis

According to Irwin's research (1990), belief in the paranormal correlated positively to fantasy proneness. Fantasy proneness has also been associated with creativity (Richards, 2009). Therefore, it is hardly surprising that Neo-shamanic practitioners, who are able to perceive and believe in the viability of phenomena not readily perceived in the normal waking state of consciousness, would express elements of paranormal belief, fantasy proneness, creativity, and sleep paralysis. The common denominator here is imagination, which the *APA Dictionary of Psychology* defines as "the faculty that produces ideas and images in the absence of direct sensory data" (VandenBos, 2015, p. 525) such as those experienced in a shamanic journey.

The 2017 study of six Neo-shamanic practitioners included anecdotal personal reports from the participants that could be interpreted as evidence of this correlation. Two of the six participants recounted incidents of sleep paralysis involving spirit entities during their interviews. One described being attacked by two Native American spirit entities who tried to rip her unborn child from her body while she was recovering from gall bladder surgery. Another participant recalled a childhood incident in which a dark, dangerous man began talking to her from outside a window. Hufford (2005) stated that individuals experiencing dramatic incidents of sleep paralysis commonly believe them to be spiritual in origin. The presence of threatening disembodied entities also appears to be a common theme among reported cases. Hinton, Hufford, and Kirmayer (2005) determined that there are both biological and intrinsic cultural beliefs at play that create a sense of unspeakable horror and danger to the dreamer. Cheyne (1982) found that themes of threat and assault were prevalent during episodes of sleep disturbance. All of these findings would be applicable in the two incidents described by the participants in the 2017 study. Revonsuo's (2009) Threat Simulation Theory of nightmares might also be applied to such occurrences such as those reported by the women in this study. The threatening invasion of a dangerous strange man in the home of a child with her parents present and an attempt by Native American men to rip an unborn child from its mother's womb are simultaneously primal, biological, and cultural. Both participants believed these events to be spiritual in nature and significant in their lives. It is possible that they were also rooted in their own personal histories based on the information revealed in their interviews.

The limbic system (the amygdala in particular) is especially active during sleep and journeys. According to McNamara (2004), the mediating hippocampus is shut down in the sleep state, while it remains active in the journey state (Winkelman, 2010). This makes it less likely that terrifying and threatening images and situations would be perceived during a journey which is focused and allows the free will of the practitioner to be utilized. Neo-shamanic practitioners frequently possess strong imaginary visualization capabilities and belief in paranormal phenomena which are in full play albeit within self-directed boundaries during journeys. The phenomena and events reported by the participants in the 2017 study are consistent with these observations. The narratives contain elements of the fantastic, including conversations with animals, trees, spirit entities, and angels that provided instructions concerning how to help preserve the environment and heal influenza. These reports are not inconsistent with those of other Neo-shamanic practitioners (Harner, 2014; Wallis, 2003).

Irwin (1990) determined that paranormal belief and fantasy proneness were connected based on his study of 92 adults. This raises the question as to whether or not Neo-shamanic practitioners (or indigenous, traditional shamans) are fantasy-prone individuals. Lynn and Rhue (1986) conducted studies on adults that determined that fantasy proneness was consistently found in creative, imaginative people with a strong ability to produce mental imagery and who held a belief in psi and anomalous phenomena. An earlier study of 27 adult women by Wilson and Barber (1982) with a high degree of hypnotizability was also found to be fantasy-prone. The women in the 1982 study demonstrated abilities as healers, telepaths, creators of vivid imagery, and recalling childhood and other memories in minute detail. The attributes of the subjects in these two studies were very similar to those displayed by the six participants in the current study. This again raises questions as to the overall fantasy proneness of contemporary Western Neo-shamanic practitioners in general.

The influence of fantasy proneness in creating a new life narrative appeared in some of the 2017 study's participants' interviews and journeys. In two instances, it translated into the autobiographical reconstruction and reframing of unhappy or traumatic events in a more meaningful evolutionary context (McAdams, 2012). Both of these women grew up in abusive home environments and endured the presence of physical, sexual, and emotional abuse as well as sudden violent death. In instances such as these, fantasy proneness became a factor in the development of a spiritual identity in keeping with MacDonald's research (2012). It must be noted that re-invention of identity through spiritual practice contains the risk of spiritual bypassing if it is not integrated into the individual's total self-perception, and the traumatizing events recognized and reconciled psychologically. The consistency of these findings implies that there likely exists a direct relationship between fantasy proneness and Neo-shamanic practice.

Intensified Schizotypy

Schizotypy is defined in the *DSM-V* (2013) as a steady pattern of eccentric behaviors and "sensory distortions" (p. 655) which undermines an individual's ability to interact, empathize, and connect in a positive manner with other people. Symptoms include unusual beliefs, magical thinking, perception of anomalous phenomena and experiences, social anxiety, and personal eccentricities in dress, lifestyle, and habits. In keeping with the previous discussion about the pitfalls of cultural dissonance, the *DSM-V* specifically refers to "Odd beliefs … that influence(s) behavior and is inconsistent with subcultural norms…" (p. 655). Were the clinical symptoms of schizotypy listed in the *DSM-V* to be presented as statements on a questionnaire, it is likely that a good many Neo-shamanic practitioners would agree that they exhibit at least three and maybe more of them. Journeying into unseen realms, interacting with the spirit world including nature spirits, spirit teachers, and ancestors, retrieving soul fragments and evicting intruding and possessing spirit entities, and even crossing the veil of death only to return are hardly consistent with contemporary Western cultural norms and mores. This raises the question "Are Neo-shamanic practitioners schizotypal?" The answer is both "yes" and "no" because Neo-shamanism is a belief system and practice that is dissonant with our culture and operates outside of the boundaries of our materialistic, rational, positivist paradigm.

According to the *DSM-V* (2013), schizotypy is classified as part of the schizophrenia spectrum. However, the *DSM* differentiates between someone exhibiting schizotypal tendencies and someone who presents as a full-blown schizophrenic (pp. 588–589). Mohr and Claridge (2015) conducted research into studies on schizotypy from which they made the determination that not only do schizotypal thoughts and tendencies occur in the general population, but that their presence can be associated with improved well-being and cognition, enhanced creativity and strong problem-solving abilities. Other research indicated that people with inherited risk for schizophrenia would seem to have a genetic advantage where creativity is concerned (Richards, 2001). Claridge (2001) recognized that spiritual awakenings and experiences are frequently interpreted to be psychotic in nature because of the similarity of symptoms. Likewise, an individual undergoing kundalini awakening can appear to be in acute psychosis from the standpoint of contemporary culture (House, 2001; Krishna, 1971). Ecstatic religious or spiritual experiences such as those described in the Bible, e.g., St. Paul on the road to Damascus, or kundalini awakenings are examples of phenomena that are pathologized when they occur outside of their original cultural contexts. This takes us back to the issue of cultural dissonance and the pathological interpretation of behaviors and/or reported experiences by observers operating within the boundaries of our cultural beliefs. But they are not necessarily pathological.

Winkelman (2004, 2010) explained that the shamanic technology required that the journey be undertaken (a) at the free will and self-determination of the practitioner and (b) with a distinct and well-articulated purpose for the journey clearly set. This separates Neo-shamanic experiences from those of visionaries who experience the numinous without desire or warning (as in the reports of the first perceivers of Marian apparitions) or of those spontaneously thrust into the transformational chaos of a kundalini awakening. But we must keep in mind that Neo-shamanism is a spiritual technology that may carry with it some attitudes and behaviors that mimic schizotypy or psychosis. On the other hand, shamanic experiences can appear to mimic a controlled schizophrenic episode and risk being judged to be pathological by doctors and therapists who are unfamiliar with the technology and worldview of Neo-shamanic practice. Repeated shamanic journeys and experiences—like kundalini and confrontation with the numinous—are the vectors of an awakening of perception of phenomena beyond the boundaries of sensory cognition. These might result in the adoption of eccentric behavior and modified behaviors that could appear to be schizotypal. It is up to the practitioner and his or her support group to determine if the behaviors are escalating to a level that render the individual unable to function normally, enjoy the pleasures of the material world, and interact with others in a positive and socially acceptable manner.

Conclusion

In general, any practice that modifies one's perception of themselves and the world around them, and in particular any practice that carries with it spiritual elements, contains the risk of dislodging the balance of the practitioner. The presence of some level of cultural dissonance with the dominant culture and beliefs of the twenty-first-century Western paradigm is to be expected for both Neo-shamanic practitioners and others who are seeking to discover their personal authenticity and/or spirituality. It is therefore important that (a) there is qualified supervision, (b) that there is a support group in place, and (c) that the new authentic identity is solidly in place. For the sake of balance and functionality, it is incumbent upon each practitioner to keep the channels of self-discovery open and enlist the aid of a teacher or therapist in the event that personal issues and/or traumas become triggered within the course of practice.

Based on the literature and the results of the 2017 study, we have seen that adoption of an updated and modified version of the techniques used by traditional shamans (Neo-shamanism) can have mental health benefits which enhance personal well-being despite its pitfalls. In addition, it can be a valuable tool for integrative self-discovery in appropriate circumstances. These techniques can also serve as adjunct practices when coupled with traditional psychotherapy. But Neo-shamanic techniques might also have value in the field of research. The next chapter discusses how the journey technique used by traditional shamans and Neo-shamans might have an application in a laboratory research environment as a means of gathering data for consciousness studies and exploration of anomalous phenomena and experiences.

References

American Psychiatric Association. (2013). *Diagnostic and statistical manual of mental disorders, 5th edition: DSM-5*. Alexandria, VA: American Psychiatric Association.

Armstrong, T. (2010). *The power of neurodiversity: Unleashing the advantage of your differently wired brain*. Cambridge, MA: Da Capo Press.

Cheyne, J. (1982). Sleep paralysis and the structure of waking nightmare hallucinations. *Dreaming, 13*(3), 163–179.

Clarke, P., Giordano, A., Cashwell, C., & Lewis, T. (2013). The straight path to healing: Using motivational interviewing to address spiritual bypass. *Journal of Counseling and Development, 91,* 87–94.

Claridge, G. (2001). Spiritual experience: Healthy psychoticism? In I. Clarke (Ed.), *Psychosis and spirituality: Exploring the New Frontier* (pp. 90–106). Philadelphia, PA: Whurr Publishers.

Eliade, M. (1964). *Shamanism: Archaic techniques of ecstasy.* Princeton, NJ: Princeton University Press.

Erikson, E. (1980). *Identity and the life cycle.* New York, NY: W.W. Norton.

Fox, J., Cashwell, C., & Picciotto, G. (2017). The opiate of the masses: Measuring spiritual bypass and its relationship to spirituality, religion, mindfulness, psychological distress and personality. *Spirituality in Clinical Practice, 4*(4), 274–287.

Harner, M. (1982). *The way of the shaman.* New York, NY: Bantam.

Harner, M. (2014). *Cave and cosmos.* Berkeley, CA: North Atlantic.

Hinton, D., Hufford, D., & Kirmayer, L. (2005). Culture and sleep paralysis. *Transcultural Psychiatry, 42*(1), 5–10.

House, R. (2001). Psychopathology, psychosis and the kundalini: Postmodern perspectives on unusual subjective experience. In I. Clarke (Ed.), *Psychosis and spirituality: Exploring the New Frontier* (pp. 107–125). Philadelphia, PA: Whurr Publishers.

Hufford, D. (2005). Sleep paralysis and spiritual experience. *Transcultural Psychiatry, 42*(1), 46–77.

Irwin, H. (1990). Fantasy proneness and paranormal beliefs. *Psychological Reports, 66*(2), 655–658.

Kjellgren, A., & Erickson, K. (2013). Methoxetamine (MXE)—A phenomenological study of experiences induced by a "legal high" from the internet. *Journal of Psychoactive Drugs, 45*(3), 276–286. https://doi.org/10.1080/02791072.2013.803647.

Kremer, J. (2004). (Post) modern brain—Shaman's brain: Evolutionary perspectives on shamanic processes and potentials. In D. Eigner (Ed.), *Consciousness: Cultural and therapeutic perspectives* (pp. 47–75). Frankfurt am Main, DE: Peter Lang International.

Krippner, S. (2000). The epistemologies and technologies of shamanic states of consciousness. *Journal of Consciousness Studies, 7,* 93–118.

Krishna, G. (1971). *Kundalini: The evolutionary energy in man.* Boston, MA: Shambhala Publications.

Lynn, S., & Rhue, J. (1986). The fantasy-prone person: Hypnosis, imagination, and creativity. *Journal of Personality and Social Psychology, 51*(2), 404–408.

MacDonald, D. (2012). Spiritual identity: Individual perspectives. In S. Schwartz, K. Luyckx, & V. Vignoles (Eds.), *Handbook of identity theory and research* (Vol. 2, pp. 531–562). New York, NY: Springer.
Masters, A. (2010). *Spiritual bypassing: When spirituality disconnects us from what really matters.* Berkeley, CA: North Atlantic.
McAdams, D. (2012). Narrative identity. In S. Schwartz, K. Luyckx, & V. Vignoles (Eds.), *Handbook of identity theory and research* (Vol. 1, pp. 99–115). New York, NY: Springer.
McClenon, J. (1997). Shamanic healing, human evolution and the origin of religion. *Journal for the Scientific Study of Religion, 36*(3), 345–354.
McClenon, J. (2011). A community survey of psychological symptoms: Evaluating evolutionary theories regarding shamanism and schizophrenia. *Mental Health, Religion & Culture, 15*(8), 799–816.
McKinnon, C. (2012). *Shamanism and spirituality in therapeutic practice.* London, UK: Singing Dragon.
McNamara, P. (2004). *An evolutionary psychology of sleep and dreams.* Westport, CT: Praeger.
Mohr, C., & Claridge, G. (2015). Schizotypy—Do not worry, it is not all worrisome. *Schizophrenia Bulletin, 4*(2), S436–S443.
Pekala, R. J. (1991). *Quantifying consciousness: Emotions, personality, and psychotherapy.* Boston, MA: Springer.
Polimeni, J. (2012). *Shamans among us: Schizophrenia, shamanism and the evolutionary origins of religion.* Sao Paulo, Brazil: Evo.
Revonsuo, A. (2009). What is an altered state of consciousness? *Philosophical Psychology, 22*(2), 187.
Richards, R. (2001). Creativity and the schizophrenic spectrum: More and more interesting. *Creativity Research Journal, 13*(1), 111–132.
Richards, R. (2009). Everyday creativity and psychopathology. *Psychological Inquiry, 4*(3), 212–217.
Richards, R., & Kinney, D. (1990). Mood swings and creativity. *Creativity Research Journal, 3*(3), 202–217.
Rock, A., & Baynes, P. (2005). Shamanic journeying imagery, constructivism, and the affect of bridge technique. *Anthropology of Consciousness, 16*(2), 50–71.
Rock, A., & Krippner, S. (2008a). Is a realistic interpretation of shamanic non-physical worlds logically incoherent? *Transpersonal Psychology Review, 12*(2), 23–31.
Rock, A., & Krippner, S. (2008b). Proposed criteria for the necessary conditions for shamanic journeying inquiry. *Journal of Scientific Exploration, 22*(2), 215–226.
Rock, A., & Krippner, S. (2008c). Some rudimentary problems pertaining to the construction of an ontology and epistemology of shamanic journeying imagery. *International Journal of Transpersonal Psychology, 27,* 12–19.

Rock, A., Abbott, G., Childargushi, H., & Kiehne, M. (2008). The effects of shamanic like stimulus conditions and the cognitive-perceptual factor of schizotypy on phenomenology. *North American Journal of Psychology, 10*(1), 79–98.

Stevens, A., & Price, J. (2006). *Evolutionary psychology: A new beginning* (2nd ed.). New York, NY: Routledge.

Thurber, J. (2016). *The secret life of Walter Mitty*. New York, NY: Penguin Press.

VandenBos, G. (Ed.). (2015). *APA dictionary of psychology* (2nd ed.). Washington, DC: American Psychological Association.

Wallis, R. (2003). *Shamans/neo-shamans: Ecstasy, alternative archaeologies, and contemporary paganism*. London, UK: Routledge.

Walsh, R. (1992). *The spirit of shamanism*. Los Angeles, CA: Jeremy P. Tarcher Inc.

Welwood, J. (1979). Principles of inner work: Psychological and spiritual. *The Journal of Transpersonal Psychology, 16*(1), 63–73.

Wilson, S., & Barber, T. (1982). The fantasy-prone personality: Implications for understanding imagery, hypnosis, and parapsychological phenomena. *PSI Research, 1*(3), 94–116.

Winkelman, M. (2004). Shamanism as the original neurotheology. *Zygon, 39*(1), 193–217.

Winkelman, M. (2009). Shamanism and the origins of spirituality and ritual healing. *Journal for the Study of Religion, Nature & Culture, 3*(4), 458–489.

Winkelman, M. (2010). *Shamanism: A biopsychosocial paradigm of consciousness and healing* (2nd ed.). Santa Barbara, CA: Praeger.

CHAPTER 6

The Journey Technique as a Method for Consciousness Studies

Abstract This chapter examines the manner in which using recorded Neo-shamanic journeys as part of a formal research setting could provide a relatively clean phenomenological and replicable data-gathering device for psychologists studying consciousness and anomalous phenomena. The unique neuropsychology of the shamanic journey enables someone in the journey state to perceive anomalous phenomena while simultaneously retaining focus and relative control of the journey and narrate the journey out loud into a recording device as the journey unfolds. The recording provides a phenomenological account of journey phenomena and experiences usually imperceptible in normal waking consciousness prior to the data being compromised by the interpretative and meaning-making processes of the participants. This chapter presents a possible research protocol that utilizes recorded shamanic journeys in a research environment.

Keywords Neo-shamanic journey · Research protocol · Phenomenology · Data gathering · Consciousness studies · Parapsychology

K. J. Bouse, *Neo-shamanism and Mental Health*,
https://doi.org/10.1007/978-3-030-31911-3_6

There is only one search: wandering…no dogma and no heresy. —Rumi

The study of consciousness presents a challenge to psychological researchers because the phenomena it produces are not contained within the positivist paradigm that directs scientific study. The phenomena that arguably signify that consciousness actually exists defy consistent observation and replication and are rarely measurable and even less likely to be predictive. Researchers have attempted to apply the standard scientific paradigm to consciousness studies as early as the 1950s at Duke University and the dream studies project that took place later at the Maimonides Medical Center in New York City. The Institute for Noetic Sciences in Petaluma, California, has done valuable research into *psi* phenomena such as telekinesis, distance viewing, and ESP through the application of traditional protocols in controlled laboratory environments which produced quantifiable results. But the vast majority of phenomena that entice consciousness researchers as potential evidence of non-material existence are non-compliant with the necessary positivist underpinnings of standard scientific inquiry. The major challenges to more inclusive research of non-material phenomena are (1) non-replication and (2) dependence on qualitative methods. In other words, the appearance and behavior of these phenomena cannot be controlled and/or reproduced dependably in a laboratory setting, and the introduction of the human element compromises any phenomenological account due to personal interpretative matrices that necessarily render any human account subjective and contaminated.

Neo-Shamanism as an Element in Consciousness Studies

Might the Neo-shamanic technology of journeying based on willed alteration of consciousness in order to perceive non-material phenomena present a potential tool for consciousness research?

Based on the literature, Neo-shamanism is a magic-based technique connecting contemporary anomalous practices of interfacing with the non-embodied entities and anomalous phenomena within the mystical and magical frameworks of the archaic past from which traditional shamanism originated (Winkelman & Baker, 2010). These beliefs include immanent divinity, the presence of the sacred in all things, Earth-centeredness, veracity of anomalous phenomena and experiences including encounters in dreams and journeys, a magical aspect to healing, divination, and life, animism, pantheism, and the omnipresence of a spirit world indiscernible through ordinary sensory cognition inform the overall lifeworlds of both traditional shamans and Neo-shamanic practitioners (Krippner & Achterberg, 2014; McClenon, 1997; Sala, 2014; Winkelman, 2010).

Although anthropologists have provided deep insight into the world of indigenous traditional shamanism through their research, relatively little inquiry has been made into the lifeworlds and consciousness matrix of Neo-shamans. Psychological inquiry based in the study of consciousness could contribute a great deal toward our understanding of these lifeworlds and spiritual contexts, including the influences of anomalous occurrences, phenomena, and mysticism. Neo-shamanism is a contemporary emergent magical and spiritual practice embracing archaic tribal beliefs, and its practitioners regularly use the ancient technology of the journey to alter consciousness at will and with purpose in order to communicate with non-embodied entities, spirit guides, and ancestors. These beliefs and lifeworlds are widely divergent from contemporary Western cultural and religious paradigms, thus making Neo-shamanism a living, cultural anomaly that operates within our dominant culture but is not of that in culture due to its embrace and internalization of a radically different reality construct (Berger & Luckmann, 1996; Geertz, 1973). As such, Neo-shamanism presents psychologists and other social scientists with a window into human consciousness involving mysticism and magic that has been long shut in the aftermath of our collective history. Exploring the lifeworlds of contemporary Western Neo-shamans can potentially add to the research and literature on which contemporary psychological therapies are based, as well as provide a basis for the modification and/or expansion of some of the more restrictive definitions currently governing the field of mental health. The journey technique used by contemporary Neo-shamanic practitioners might itself provide a useful tool for consciousness studies because it is:

1. Replicable;
2. Workable in a controlled environment; and
3. Offers immediate access to anomalous phenomena and experiences prior to processing through the meaning-making lenses of the practitioner.

Is the Neo-Shamanic Journey an Example of Self-Hypnosis?

The *APA Dictionary of Psychology* (2015) defines self-hypnosis as "the process of putting oneself into a trance or trancelike state, typically through autosuggestion" (p. 956). This definition would certainly apply to the journey process used by traditional shamans and Neo-shamanic practitioners. Cardena and Krippner discussed the elements of self-hypnosis present in worldwide shamanic practices including the utilization of learned skills to facilitate journeying to interface with spirit entities, plant and animal spirits to acquire information and facilitate healing (Lynn & Rhue, 1986). The factors of genetic proclivity toward hypnotizability, creativity, fantasy proneness, and encounters with anomalous phenomena are common to both those in shamanic practice and what Cardena and Krippner refer to as "hypnotic virtuosos" (p. 750). The shamanic journey is a technology that requires the practitioner to willfully assume a trancelike state in order to perceive phenomena for a specific purpose, as would a skilled self-hypnotist. Contemporary Westerners have used a form of self-hypnosis to overcome bad habits, physical ailments, and emotional and psychological blockages. Shamanic practitioners incorporate elements of the sacred and service to others in their journeys. It is these two factors that separate them from others who practice self-hypnosis for self-healing. That said the two techniques are close siblings if not identical.

Neo-Shamanism as a Potential Phenomenological Protocol

Research into Neo-shamanism might potentially yield another benefit, this in the area of consciousness research. The journey technique used by Neo-shamanic practitioners has potential to be a viable method for the gathering of phenomenological data for analysis because it is a bridge between normal waking consciousness and the subconscious. The journey is the core technology of shamanic practice that has survived first hand through indigenous and traditional societies and once removed through teaching the journey technique to contemporary Westerners through workshops, classes, and seminars by academics (e.g., Michael Harner) and members of traditional cultures who are willing to teach the technology to outsiders. The journey is undertaken at the specified will and the pre-defined purpose/focus determined by the practitioner. Neuroscientific observations have revealed that during the journey, the brain is able to simultaneously use and integrate the functions of both the limbic system and the cerebral cortex in a way that enables the practitioners to narrate the journey as it unfolds (Harner, 2005; Winkelman, 2004, 2010). The significance of such narratives is their potential to create a clean qualitative phenomenological record of phenomena usually imperceptible through sensory cognition as they appear during the journey since it is possible for researchers to record the spoken narrative of the participants while they are in the journey (Harner, 2005). As such, they are less likely to be contaminated by the practitioner's post-journey filters of personal meaning-making and rationalization since the interpretative lenses of the practitioner appear to be absent or strongly reduced in the journey state. The tape-recorded narrations of participants in the journey state obtained during the course of my research demonstrated the value of such recordings in producing clean phenomenological accounts for analysis of elements such as phenomena, patterns, and synchronicities. This information can then be represented statistically in order to provide quantitative substance to results obtained by means of a controlled qualitative protocol.

Benefits of Using Recorded Journeys for Data Gathering

The primary benefits of using the recorded narratives of people in the journey state are (1) the controlled aspects of the journey, (2) lack of risk to the participants, and (3) providing a clean phenomenological database for analysis and quantitative representation. Similar phenomena might be perceived by individuals during altered states of consciousness such as those experienced during dreams, hypnogogic and hypnopompic states, lucid dreaming, guided visualizations, channeling, meditation, and self-hypnosis. However, the shamanic journey is a state of consciousness that is differentiated from these other non-waking states by a combination of characteristics that make it very promising for application as part of a research protocol. These characteristics are:

- The journey state is entered into at the will of the practitioner.
- It is approached from a state of normal waking consciousness with specific purpose, direction, and focus.
- The practitioner knows specifically how to direct the journey to a specific destination (e.g., the Lower World or the Upper World) for the specific purpose of the journey.

- The practitioner is trained in journey work and is knowledgeable of protocols and protective strategies necessary when interfacing with the world of the spirits.
- Neo-shamans use repetitive, rhythmic drumming to shift into the appropriate state of consciousness and drive their journeys (Harner, 1982; Rock & Krippner, 2011). This eliminates the need for drugs, fasting, sleep deprivation, and other methods of consciousness alteration frequently used by traditional shamans in indigenous settings. The relative safety of the drumming technique is desirable for research work because of the reduced risk to the participants, its controlled replication through pre-recording, adaptability to a research setting, and ability of the research team to modify variables such as duration and volume of drumming. It is important to note that repetitive drumming can trigger seizures in people with epilepsy. Such seizure-prone individuals should avoid using drumming as a means of consciousness alteration.
- The practitioner maintains some rationality and function, sense of purpose, and control over the journey and has self-determination over his/her actions during the journey.
- The practitioner in the journey state has the ability to ask questions and converse with spirit entities encountered during the journey. They can simultaneously narrate orally what they perceive in the journey as it unfolds and they are deep in the journey state (Harner, 2005).
- The practitioner can change locations within the journey and abort the journey at will.
- According to Winkelman (2004, 2010), laboratory experiments on shamans in the journey state revealed that both the limbic system and the cerebral cortex were engaged and integrated in a manner which enabled the participants to perceived phenomena that were imperceptible during normal waking consciousness (Rock & Krippner, 2011) while maintaining the rational and verbal function of the executive brain.
- Taped journey narratives produced while the participant is in the journey state provide clear, rich reports of what the participants are perceiving and experiencing during the journey as it happens.

What Can the Content of Journeys Potentially Tell Us About Consciousness?

Journeys are very much like films in that they contain an overlapping of the specific and the semiotic. This immediately brings up the question of whether or not the person taking the journey acts as the journey's *auteur*. Research into the origins and production of journey phenomena (Rock & Baynes, 2005, 2007; Rock & Casey, 2005; Rock & Krippner 2008a, 2008b, 2008c) indicated that there is a definite correlation between the phenomena perceived in the journey state and the personal matrix of the voyager (Bouse, 2017). This is particularly true of contemporary Neo-shamanic practitioners since they have developed highly individualized life-worlds based on biology, personal history, ethnicity, culture, and spiritual orientation as opposed to shamans in traditional societies whose beliefs and practices are integral elements of the surrounding societal worldview and culture. The specific phenomena observed and experienced in the journey as being immediately relevant to the question/focus of the journey are more than likely to be straightforward and easily traced to the personal and cultural contexts of the person experiencing the journey. This was evidenced by the journey excerpts recorded during the 2017 study. These phenomena are frequently reflections of the contextual lenses of a given participant during the journey a priori of any subsequent meaning-making process and interpretation by the participant. An example of this would be the following journey excerpt from one of the 2017 study participants who spent much of her life in urban environments:

> I ask eagle for his help in being able to help someone heal from influenza. As we cover the ground flying over the stark frozen land an image of my spirit teacher, a kind looking woman with flowing white blonde hair comes along side us. She's on a broom like a Hallowe'en witch this time. Then she's just flying along with us. We start to see tall buildings, beautifully built, nice architecture. And then we veer away from those to the right and begin to see mountains and rolling hills, beautiful green below us.

Based on the biographical information this participant provided during the interview, there would appear to be a strong element of replication between the imagery encountered in the journey and the imagery she has encountered in her normal, waking state. The spirit teacher she reported seeing was reflective of a fairly common cultural image: The archetype of the witch or wise woman is common in contemporary Western culture and frequently is a symbol of arcane, esoteric knowledge and powers.

But do journey phenomena merely reflect the contextual lenses of the participant? As with dreams, a portion of the reported imagery and phenomenology mirrors the reality constructs and personal matrices of the individual taking the journey. Yet there are situations wherein such mirroring seems to be absent, and the reported imagery does not have a correlative relationship to anything that is in the personal matrix of the participant. The recorded narration by one of the 2017 participants exemplifies such a parade of anomalous imagery:

> We're on a brown plain. Seems pretty lifeless. The word "devastation" is in my mind. Turning to the right and walking away from the river. There's something – might be ice, like the end of a glacier. A waterfall that froze. It's ice. And there're some metal steps. One side of them is coming out of the frozen area, but there's room enough to walk up the steps. The first one was high up. I had to crawl up on the elephant's back to reach the first step. So we start to climb barefoot. The steps are cold. There're some flying creatures. Heads look kind of like sparklers or dandelion heads. Dandelion seeds. Look inside. There's like a glass globe inside. So I'd like to go inside there. And just start to climb in. Animals come too. We're all pretty small but we fit. We might be inside a speck of pollen – the color amber. I'm getting uncomfortable in here. There's a dragon who has been trapped inside. There're dragon tears. Has long, long hair, like old long gray hair. He'd like to come out but he's scared to leave. We can open it up. He thinks it might be poisonous for him outside of the bubble. So when he got scared he started to heat up, and that was the way to break out of the bubble and to be released outdoors. He thought the poison was…it was horrifying. We had to calm down. He wanted to escape but he thought it would kill him. Meanwhile the rest of us just want to get out of there and bring him out too.

There are considerable phenomenological differences between the journey accounts of these two participants which are particularly striking when one considers that both journeys were focused on finding an answer to the questions "What can I do to help preserve and protect the local environment?" The recorded narrative by this participant brings to mind paintings by Hieronymus Bosch (bubbles, glass globes, dandelion heads that only look like dandelion heads but are portals to the interior of the bubble) interspersed with allusions to ancient archetypal images, e.g., the Earth power as a dragon (Celtic and Germanic). Without going into an intricate inventory and analysis of the images recounted, it is obvious that this participant has encountered phenomena originating from an area of consciousness far removed from the mundane world. It is journeys and accounts such as this one that offer us possible glimpses into shared consciousness, genetic memory, and the supernormal and anomalous phenomena—into the very nature of consciousness itself. A journey such as this one gives us access to the alien and unknown in much the same way that an astronaut landing on a distant planet does. It is these reported phenomena that have the potential to provide researchers with seeds for further study and analysis as they seek a better understanding of the scope and nature of human consciousness.

An interesting point is that when these same two participants journeyed to find the answer to the question "What is the best way to heal someone who is suffering from severe influenza?" they both received the answer that the mashed and brewed bark of the (local) tulip poplar tree reduced pain, inflammation, and fever. These two people have extremely different lifeworlds, and the second one quoted here has a much longer history of Neo-shamanic practice than the first. And yet they received the same answer to the same question, which makes one wonder "where did the answer come from?" One further point of interest is that while the second voyager received the message about tulip poplar bark aurally, the first woman saw the bark plainly as well as how to prepare it. She did not know that it was tulip poplar until she performed a Google search of common indigenous deciduous trees of the local area and was able to recognize the bark she saw distinctly in her journey identified as tulip poplar through her online search.

The other participants described their journey phenomena within the contexts of their personal filters, e.g., Christian (Protestant), Christian (Roman Catholic), and New Age. Their journeys were highly personal in nature, but shared the narrative that their spirit teacher(s) showed them a holographic image of a "patient" and showed them how to heal that "patient" energetically using light, air, and focused cleansing energy. Four of the participants received the same answer to the question "What can I personally do to preserve and protect the local environment?" These answers all reportedly came from animal spirits and directed the voyagers to take care of the water, trees, and the vegetation. Therefore, it would appear that:

a. Journeys and perceived images and phenomena by Neo-shamanic practitioners reflect individual lifeworlds.
b. The voyagers frequently reported similar answers to focus questions despite semiotic discrepancies in the imagery.
c. The information as narrated by the practitioners in the journey state appears to have been presented to the individual practitioners in a manner that facilitated their understanding of the information regardless of variances in personal contexts.
d. Some perceived journey phenomena are completely anomalous to personal and cultural influences.

According to an article that was recently published (Mayer, 2013) in *Science Alert*, a group of scientists at Emory University researching the potential efficacy of old herbal remedies in overcoming current pharmaceutical challenges discovered that the bark of the tulip poplar and white oak possessed properties that dismantled the defensive sheath of the strain of *Staphylococcus* responsible for MRSA—a so-called superbug that appears to be impervious to known antibiotics. The Emory team learned of the medicinal attributes of the tulip poplar (and other local plants) from the field notes of Dr. Frances Porcher—a physician in the Confederate Army during the American Civil War. Two participants in the 2017 study received the message during their journeys about healing influenza through the use of tulip poplar bark. It's is interesting not only that two diverse practitioners accessed the identical information to a specific question, but also that the information obtained through their journeys was verified by medical researchers in the lab. What might this tell us about the transpersonal nature of consciousness and the potential value of Neo-shamanism as a viable contemporary adjunct to healing protocols?

Protocol Template

The following is a protocol that developed from the original research design for the 2017 study of the lifeworlds of Neo-shamanic practitioners. It represents a potential method for using shamanic journey technology in a controlled laboratory setting in order to create a phenomenological library of images and experiences that can become a database for analysis and further inquiry in consciousness research. Based on the results of the 2017 study, the application of a protocol such as the one outlined below holds promise.

Rationale

Neo-shamanic practitioners employ the same journey technique as many traditional shamans in order to gain insight and information, facilitate healing, and assist in the process of death. The journey state requires a definitive purpose and/or question, and the journey is initiated at will from a normal waking state of consciousness. During the journey, the practitioner's limbic system and cerebral cortex are working simultaneously (Winkelman, 2010) so that the journey can be narrated as it unfolds. By using identical sensory deprivation devices, e.g., blindfold, quiet, darkened room, and listening to repetitive rhythmic drumming through earbuds, it is possible for the voyager to report what he/she is seeing and experiencing while in the journey state by narrating occurrences and images into a recording device. This technique was developed by Dr. Sandra Harner (2005) to aid in psychotherapy. But rather than allowing the participant to integrate and interpret the meaning of the journey upon its conclusion, the desired result is a clear phenomenological record for analysis. The resultant phenomenological journey records and subsequent data analyses have the potential to present researchers with a snapshot of areas of consciousness existing beyond but simultaneously with normal waking consciousness and sensory-based cognition.

Research Questions

The major question is: What is the nature and landscape of expanded consciousness? Subsidiary questions are:

1. What can the phenomena encountered during journeys tell us about expanded consciousness that we do not already know?
2. How much of the perceived phenomena are:
    - Personal
    - Cultural
    - Archetypal
    - Anomalous
3. How do these phenomena tally up with global mythologies and religions?
4. What does the information collected in journeys tell us about universality of consciousness?

5. How do journeys differ phenomenologically among practitioners?
6. How consistent is the information received by multiple practitioners during journeys?
7. What is the ratio of verifiable to unverifiable information? Is the information received relevant to transpersonal understanding and/or everyday existence?

Screening Participants

A study like this requires careful screening of participants to insure the highest possibility of clean and equitable results. Initially, all participants need to fall within US National Institutes of Health Guidelines to eliminate participation by potentially at-risk individuals. Substance abusers or people on prescribed psychoactive or opioid medications would be considered "at-risk" for the purposes of this research. For the safety of the participants, anyone wishing to participate who is working with a mental health professional would be required to have (a) permission from that professional and (b) agreement of the professional to be available in the event of a crisis resulting from the journey work involved.

All participants selected for this study would attend an orientation session to understand their rights under law as participants in a study, the procedure of the study including expectations of them, their rights to withdraw from the study completely or not participate in any given session for their own reasons, and review and sign letters stating full disclosure, informed consent, and confidentiality. This is in compliance with the Code of Ethics of the American Psychological Association and the guidelines of the National Institutes of Health of the United States.

It would be beneficial to the quality of the research if the participants were screened as part of the selection process. Potential participants should be interviewed and answer questionnaires to determine the lenses through which they view themselves and the world which could have influence on their phenomena they perceive and the flavor of the journeys they would undertake. Additionally, it would be advisable for the candidates to undertake diagnostic testing for fantasy proneness and schizotypy to ensure that they fall within a desirable predetermined range in order to reduce the potential for false narratives and contrived accounts. All participants should be allowed to work with a researcher with knowledge and experience in Neo-shamanic journey protocols in order to ensure that they are able to employ the journey technique successfully within the research protocol and are able to narrate the journey as it takes place. Such standardization—while potentially not optimal to some Neo-shamanic practitioners—would be valuable in optimizing replication potential in a controlled setting.

Ideally, participants in this study would be:

- Between 30 and 65 years of age.
- Do not have a history of heavy drug or alcohol use.
- Have no criminal record.
- Have a minimum of a completed secondary education.
- Have no dangerous physical health conditions or are undertaking a serious pharmaceutical protocol, e.g., chemotherapy.
- Have no past history of serious mental health problems, e.g., borderline personality, bipolar, severe depression, schizophrenia, and antisocial disorder.
- Well grounded in the mundane world through job, family, friends, and have a strong support system in place.
- Are either inexperienced at journeying or have very limited exposure to it.
- Are not subject to seizures and epilepsy.

Interviews provide researchers with insight and information regarding the contextual matrices of the participants. All interviews should be recorded and transcribed. When presented with clear open-ended questions and a person-centered reflective approach to inquiry, participants are encouraged to explore themselves deeply in the course of responding (Carkhuff, 2009). This technique can yield rich information that can help define the reality constructs of the participant which is an important element in data analysis. The questions used from the Interview Questionnaire (Appendix 5 in Chapter 2) in the 2017 study proved to evoke deep responses and provide much insight into the lifeworld of the participants.

Questionnaires covering specific areas of belief such as those used in the 2017 study (Appendices 1–4 in Chapter 2) are useful tools in determining key elements of the lifeworlds, reality constructs, core beliefs, and values of the participants. Questionnaires focusing on spiritual orientation, past personal history, belief in the supernormal, and cultural influence would be relevant as part of this protocol in order to get a baseline on each participant which could be useful in the analysis of the data. Questionnaires are particularly useful in establishing an in-depth database of individual life-worlds specific to the research that can augment the information gleaned from the interviews. This individual knowledge of each participant's matrix becomes important in the determination of which reported phenomena are anomalous to their acknowledged beliefs, previous experiences, and expectations. During the 2017 study, it was useful to identify consistencies and incongruities within the reported journey phenomena and the beliefs and attitudes individuals revealed on the questionnaires. The same goes for interview answers. Finally, the information on questionnaires is easily quantifiable and not quite as subjective in nature as responses to questions in an interview.

Tests are another way to not only provide quantifiable results, but also assist in determining a prospective participant's proclivities toward schizotypy, fantasy proneness, involvement of imagination in everyday life, and creativity. The American Psychological Association has a series of tests that are self-reporting questionnaires that address these topics. These include the Creative Experiences Questionnaire (Merckelbach, Horselenberg, & Muris, 2001), the Imaginative Involvement Questionnaire, the Schizotypy Experimental Questionnaire, the Anomalous Experiences Inventory, and the Revised Transliminality Scale. Tests such as these could provide information that might identify situations in which participation in a project such as this might be detrimental to the participant, e.g., exaggerated schizotypal tendencies or possible contaminate the journey narratives with false reports which might be the case with someone who is excessively fantasy prone.

Setting

The journeys should all occur in the same place, which should be quiet, safe, neutral, and comfortable. The researcher should be able to control the lighting so that it is soothing and warm, and there should be minimal interruptive sounds from outside the room such as traffic or human conversation. Ideally the setting should be a small sitting room with a comfortable couch and rug so that the participant can have the option of lying on the couch or stretching out on the floor. Each participant should have his or her own pair of earbuds or headphones that they can connect to the CD player or other audio device so that they can hear the drumming recording. Participants should be comfortable with the microphone hooked to the device recording their journey narratives on their chests or collars so that their narratives will be clear and easily transcribed. This procedure requires that electrical outlets are accessible without the use of extension cords. The researcher can adjust the volume of the drumming CD at the direction of the participant. Water and protein snacks would ideally be on hand, as it is frequently helpful for voyagers to eat something to help them ground after their journeys. This is particularly important if the participants are driving after the session.

The researchers should have one or two therapists on call during the course of the research in the event that a journey triggers a traumatic or spiritual crisis in a participant. These therapists should be open-minded to the research and experienced at helping someone work through nightmares, anomalous experiences, or spiritual crises.

Procedure

All of the journeys should be undertaken on a strictly individual and confidential basis. There should ideally be between 6 and 12 participants. The sessions should be held at weekly intervals and should be allotted no less than an hour and no more than an hour and a half. All participants will attend a daylong workshop during which time they will have the project orientation, explanation, and learn the basics of journey technique.

1. Have the participant complete a short intake questionnaire to determine:
    a. How are they feeling in general?
    b. Have they had any major stressors in work or personal life within the past 2 days?
    c. Did they have any problems traveling to the research site?
    d. Have they had any health complaints within the past 2 days?
    e. Are they on any kind of medication either prescription or OTC?
    f. Have they had any outstanding dreams and/or nightmares since the last session?
    g. Is there anything that is preying on their mind currently?
2. Make sure that the participant is 100% comfortable as they lay down and that all blindfolds, recording, and listening devices are operational

and comfortable to the participant. Remind the participant to narrate the journey as it unfolds.

3. Dim the light and ask the participant to take three deep breaths. State the direction and intent of the journey to the participant, e.g., "I am going to the (upper/lower) world to seek out my (teacher/animal spirits) to find out (state the question)." Repeat this three times.
4. Begin the drumming CD. (Note: These journeys should only be 5–7 minutes in length).
5. Researcher should sit quietly and take notes during the journey. They should follow the journey narration and be prepared to interrupt the journey and stop the journey CD if the participant begins to show signs of distress and seems unable to stop the journey themselves.
6. When the journey is completed, brighten the room, unhook the participant from the devices, and offer them water and a snack. Discuss the journey with the participant to help them to integrate it, and make some sense of what they just saw and experienced. Participants might appreciate the chance to write down their journeys in a notebook or to draw the images they perceived. It is always good to have paper, crayons, and pens available for their use.
7. Ensure that the participant is stable and alert before they leave. Offer them a transcript of the journey once it is made, and arrange for the next session.

Data Gathering

The means of data gathering is transcribing the recorded narratives of the journeys. There should be six journey sessions at the rate of one per week for six weeks with each session covering one question. Each session should be 60–90 minutes in length. The sessions can be scheduled in such a way that the participants move through the questions at their own pace depending on their schedules. The questions devised should be general and non-personal in nature to minimize the potential for triggering trauma or repressed issues for the participants and to be in keeping with the shamanic tradition of helping the community.

Assessment

The first step in assessment is the transcription of the narrations. This narration should provide a clean non-interpreted phenomenological record. Elements of the journey can be broken down into broad categories including images, experiences, sounds, landscapes, and activities. As in dreamwork, the individual phenomena can be further described as to what they said, did, appeared, and the feelings invoked in the participants. The journey phenomena can be further assessed within the context of each individual participant:

- Are the images consistent from journey to journey?
- Do the phenomena ever appear to behave incongruously?
- Which phenomena elicited positive responses in the participant? Negative? Neutral?
- Did the journey answer the focus question? If so, how?
- Which journey images are consistent with the lifeworld of the participant based on the information recorded on the questionnaires and interview responses?
- Which journey images are anomalous to the lifeworld and previous journey experience of any given participant?
- What are the similarities of phenomena encountered across the field of participants?
- Which phenomena stand out as anomalous or especially significant?

The phenomena themselves are the data and can be analyzed in any way that assists the researchers in answering the questions stated above about the nature of consciousness. One of the primary areas of inquiry is the origin of the phenomena—whether they are the products of the memories and lifeworld of a participant, or did they have a transpersonal genesis.

Pitfalls of Journey Phenomena as Scientific Accounts

Despite the screening and testing, the research is dependent upon the truthful narration of the journey by the participants. It is possible for a participant to embellish or create a false narration. Such fallacies would be difficult to detect and might inadvertently be included in the phenomena database and subsequent analysis. If the narrations of a particular participant consistently seem "off" to the researcher, those narratives can always be eliminated from the data pool.

Caveats

The welfare of the participants is the responsibility of the researchers, and it is incumbent upon them to ensure that everything is done within ethical and legal guidelines and that the research conforms to the highest of professional standards. It would be in the best interest of participants and researchers if there was a research assistant in the room along with the primary researcher and participant to help if needed should an emergency arise and ensure that all professional standards and behavior are followed. Likewise, participants might be encouraged to come to the sessions in the company of a trusted friend or relative.

Conclusions

There is much that can be learned from the phenomenological content of shamanic journeys. Recording the journey narratives as they unfold provides researchers with frequently detailed and rich accounts of anomalous encounters and experiences that may provide us with windows into the nature of consciousness. Such a study is qualitative and not immune to the more commonly cited pitfalls of qualitative inquiry, but it has an intrinsic element that allows for a reasonably consistent level of control as well as improved replication. The procedure outlined above focuses on the raw phenomenal content perceived by individuals using a shamanic journey technique devoid of interpretation by the narrator. By recording the phenomena as they occur under controlled and replicable conditions, they become observable data that can be analyzed and quantified in a way that eliminates the wild card nature of most so-called anecdotal evidence which is more often tainted through a posteriori interpretation by the reporting individuals.

References

Berger, P., & Luckmann, T. (1996). *The social construction of reality: A treatise on the sociology of knowledge*. New York, NY: Anchor.

Bouse, K. (2017). *Neo-shamanism as a developmental, spiritual matrix for contemporary magical discovery and practice* (Doctoral dissertation). Available from ProQuest Dissertations and Theses database (No. 10742675).

Carkhuff, R. (2009). *The art of helping* (9th ed.). Amherst, MA: Possibilities Publishing Inc.

Geertz, C. (1973). *The interpretation of cultures*. New York, NY: Basic.

Harner, M. (1982). *The way of the shaman*. New York, NY: Bantam.

Harner, M. (2005). The history and work of the Foundation for Shamanic Studies. *Shamanism (25th Anniversary Issue)*, *18*(1–2). Available at http://www.shamanism.org/articles/article18.html.

Harner, S. (2005). Presence in existential-humanistic psychotherapy and in the shamanic journey. *International Institute for Humanistic Studies*. http://www.human-studies.com.

Krippner, S., & Achterberg, J. (2014). Anomalous healing experiences. In E. Cardena, S. Lynn, & S. Krippner (Eds.), *Varieties of anomalous experiences: Examining the scientific evidence* (2nd ed., pp. 273–302). Washington, DC: American Psychological Association.

Lynn, S., & Rhue, J. (1986). The fantasy-prone person: Hypnosis, imagination, and creativity. *Journal of Personality and Social Psychology, 51*(2), 404–408.

Mayer, G. (2013). Spirituality and extraordinary experiences: Methodological remarks and some empirical findings. *Journal of Empirical Theology, 26*(2), 188–206.

McClenon, J. (1997). Shamanic healing, human evolution and the origin of religion. *Journal for the Scientific Study of Religion, 36*(3), 345–354.

Merckelbach, H., Horselenberg, R., & Muris, P. (2001). The creative experiences questionnaire (CEQ): A brief self-report measure of fantasy proneness. *Personality and Individual Differences, 31*, 987–995.

Rock, A., & Baynes, P. (2005). Shamanic journeying imagery, constructivism, and the affect of bridge technique. *Anthropology of Consciousness, 16*(2), 50–71.

Rock, A., & Baynes, P. (2007). What are the origins of shamanic journeying imagery? The modification of hypnoanalytic technique to address and enduring methodological problem. *The Humanistic Psychologist, 35*(4), 349–361.

Rock, A., & Casey, P. (2005). Experimental study of ostensibly shamanic journeying imagery in naïve participants I: Antecedents. *Anthropology of Consciousness, 16*(2), 72–92.

Rock, A., & Krippner, S. (2008a). Is a realistic interpretation of shamanic nonphysical worlds logically incoherent? *Transpersonal Psychology Review, 12*(2), 23–31.

Rock, A., & Krippner, S. (2008b). Proposed criteria for the necessary conditions for shamanic journeying inquiry. *Journal of Scientific Exploration, 22*(2), 215–226.

Rock, A., & Krippner, S. (2008c). Some rudimentary problems pertaining to the construction of an ontology and epistemology of shamanic journeying imagery. *International Journal of Transpersonal Psychology, 27*, 12–19.

Rock, A., & Krippner, S. (2011). *Demystifying shamans and their world: An interdisciplinary study*. Charlottesville, VA: Imprint Academic.

Sala, L. (2014). *Ritual: A magical perspective*. New Delhi, IN: Nirala.

Winkelman, M. (2004). Shamanism as the original neurotheology. *Zygon, 39*(1), 193–217.

Winkelman, M. (2010). *Shamanism: A biopsychosocial paradigm of consciousness and healing* (2nd ed.). Santa Barbara, CA: Praeger.

Winkelman, M., & Baker, J. (2010). *Supernatural and natural: A biocultural approach to religion*. New York, NY: Routledge.

CHAPTER 7

Conclusions

Abstract This chapter briefly recapitulates the findings and conclusions of the preceding chapters. It postulates that further expanded research into Neo-shamans and their practice encompassing a larger participant base than the 2017 study has potential value to psychologists to understanding Neo-shamanic lifeworlds in particular and other alternative lifeworlds and spiritualities (e.g. New Age, Wiccan) in general. It explores the benefits of employing Neo-shamanic practice and skilled, professional Neo-shamanic practitioners acting as healers as adjuncts to traditional psychotherapy. Finally, it asks the question "What if?" research into the expanded lifeworlds of Neo-shamans which incorporates anomalous phenomena and experiences could result in Kuhnian paradigm shift in our cultural perception of reality.

Keywords Neo-shamanism · Psychotherapy · Alternative lifeworlds · Anomalous phenomena · Paradigm shift

K. J. Bouse, *Neo-shamanism and Mental Health*,
https://doi.org/10.1007/978-3-030-31911-3_7

Rise up nimbly and go on your strange journey. —Rumi

During the course of this book, we have explored how Neo-shamanic practice and how it has the potential to elevate one's sense of individual well-being. We have also examined how the utilization of the Neo-shamanic technique of journeying might be a promising tool in consciousness research and as part of a template for self-discovery including expanded awareness and individuation when used as part of a supervised curriculum. There has also been an overview of potential hazards present in adopting a practice and technology that lack a supporting cultural matrix such as societal dissociation, schizotypy, elevated fantasy proneness, cultural dissonance, and spiritual bypassing. These discussions were based on the successful completion of a doctoral program supervised by acknowledged experts in shamanism, creativity, and dreams, but also the observations of nearly 30 years of study, practice, and teaching Neo-shamanism which corroborated the formal results of the 2017 research study discussed in the preceding chapters. That study was focused on a small group of fairly homogenous participants in an isolated area. It would be valuable to expand those protocols to include a more diversified and widespread group of participants to determine if:

a. The results reflected the conclusions of the 2017 study?
b. If there were differences, what were they?
c. How did the collective and individual phenomena of the larger group deviate from the phenomena reported by the 2017 participants?
d. If so, what was the reason(s) for the phenomenological deviation?

From a research perspective, it would be valuable to use the results from the expanded study to strengthen the phenomenological database for further research, as well as provide insight into the reality constructs present in a larger representation of lifeworlds.

Benefits of Neo-Shamanic Technique as Psychological Adjunct

If a Neo-shamanic practice is well integrated within the individual's identity and *Dasein* as an augmented aspect of normal waking consciousness and function, it is likely to have a beneficial effect upon the well-being, creativity, and overall expanded consciousness of the practitioner. This is especially true if the practitioner utilizes shamanic techniques and skills at the request of others for information and/or healing, for such instances can indicate the presence of a supportive community of people with similar beliefs, e.g., Neo-pagans. Under such circumstances, the practitioner is operating consistently within the parameters of traditional shamanism.

Neo-shamanism holds promise as an adjunct to standard therapeutic practices. Sandra Harner's development of shamanic counseling (2005) and Christa Mackinnon's integration of integrating Neo-shamanic practice as part of psychotherapy (2012) detailed the manner in which utilization of the journey technique can be a beneficial adjunct to the therapeutic process. In addition, the techniques used by many Neo-shamans might be integrated into a well-supervised and balanced curriculum of self-discovery. But Neo-shamanic healing itself might present a useful element as part of standard therapeutic practice when applied to the treatment of conditions such as depression, schizotypy, borderline personality, anxiety, and dissociative disorders among others. It could be particularly beneficial in cases where the client holds spiritual beliefs and/or inhabits a lifeworld anomalous to that of the current cultural mainstream. Inclusion of Neo-shamanic healing in the clinical setting would require that practitioners are trained, vetted, subscribe to Codes of Ethics, and ongoing professional education in accordance with the standards applied to professional psychologists and therapists. Provided that the patient is amenable to accepting the services of a Neo-shaman based on worldview and the belief in a spiritual element to his or her psychological difficulty, incorporating Neo-shamanic healing as part of a healing psychological protocol could be valuable in the ongoing good mental health of the patient. The ability of Neo-shamanic practice to assist in the integration of physical, mental, and spiritual aspects could be particularly useful when incorporated into standard therapeutic practice, especially when it enlists the efforts of the patient in effectuating his or her own recovery.

The Shamanic View of Mental Health

In the shamanic worldview, everything is alive, sentient, and contains the spark of divinity. This is a worldview that is opposite that of our contemporary Western culture, which tends to see illness (physical and mental) as clinical manifestations of disease or disorder. Psychology developed on the medical model with a concentration on alleviating the symptoms of mental imbalance evidenced by disordered behavior in the material world to ensure the full functioning of the patient. Psychology looks to physiological issues and chemical imbalances to determine the cause of disordered behavior patterns that are causing pain to the patient and undermining his or her ability to participate fully in the life of the material world. Current practice looks toward psychotherapy and pharmaceuticals in order to bring relief to the patient in accordance with the medical model.

Mental distress in the shaman's worldview is dealt with on a spiritual level, because it follows a hermetic model in which everything manifesting in the physical world has a correlate in the spiritual world which must be addressed and resolved in order for the patient to heal. It also embraces the belief that the spirit world exists simultaneously with the material world, albeit outside of the scope of our cognitive sensory apparatus. For example, someone who exhibits a withdrawal from social contact, begins acting in an erratic and unusual manner, and speaks about hearing voices would likely be diagnosed with schizophrenia by a contemporary Western psychiatrist after any mediating cause such as alcohol or other substance abuse was eliminated. The patient would undergo intensive and lengthy psychotherapy and prescribed anti-psychotic drugs in an effort to effect recovery and return to normal life. If this same patient were part of a society that looked to shamanic practice for healing, the shaman would journey on the patient's behalf on the request of the patient and his or her family in order to determine the cause of the disturbance. It would not be unusual if the shaman would find that the patient has been possessed by a disembodied spirit of some kind such as the ghost of someone who has died but not fully reintegrated in the world beyond the material world or by an entity that wants to feed off the life force of the host (patient). In this case, the shaman would solicit the aid of his or her spirit allies to assist in either:

1. Getting the ghost to see that it needed to release the hold it has on material life through the patient and allow the shaman to escort it to where the souls of the deceased go after death in that specific culture, or
2. Prying the possessing entity away from the life force field of the patient, and sending them far away.

The shaman might also come back with instructions for rituals and nature-based remedies for the patient in order to ensure that the healing was complete and internalized by the patient. In some cases, the tribe community is asked to take steps to appease the spirits for protection for t only the patient but also the members of the group at large.

This is a form of faith healing that is based on three elements that are he core of all spirit-based healing protocols from indigenous cultures, lical accounts, and contemporary Christian faith healings. These are:

- Belief,
- Empathy, and
- Hypnosis.

These three elements must work synergistically in order to be effective regardless of the spiritual context of the healing. Belief requires that the patient believe not only that the shaman's ability to heal through interaction with the world of spirits, but also that healing through spirit is effective and will work for them. Empathy is the energetic and emotional connection of consciousness between the patient and the shaman and frequently the community (McClenon, 1997) during the healing procedure. Hypnosis is the engine that drives the healing process because everyone involved is in an altered state of consciousness to a greater or lesser degree. The hypnotic element reinforces the belief and empathy factors, which reinforce the power of the healing effort. McClenon discussed the manner in which hypnotizability was a survival trait because it brought community members together through the phenomenon of group mind and also facilitated the efficacy of the healing ritual and procedure.

While contemporary mental health professionals speak of post-traumatic stress, depression, and dissociation, Neo-shamanic practitioners consider soul loss and spirit intrusions. Psychosis is framed as possession or soul fragmentation. What would be diagnosed as an acute onset of obsessive-compulsive disorder by a contemporary Western therapist would be perceived as the intrusion of a discarnate entity in the shamanic view. A recurring dream or nightmare would not be considered as a sleep disorder as it might in today's clinician's office, but would be approached as a message from the spirits that may have significance for the person having the dreams or the community as a whole. Both the contemporary and the traditional shamanic approach have demonstrated themselves to be effective within their respective contexts. But can the shamanic approach be valid within the matrix of contemporary medicine and mental health philosophies?

Shamanic and Spiritual Healing as Therapeutic Protocols

Returning to the idea of integration of mind, body, and spirit, it would seem that the shamanic approach performed by competent and experienced Neo-shamanic practitioners would be a valuable adjunct to allopathic medicine and modern psychology despite the anomalous nature of their practices. Shamanic healing is like any other kind of spiritual healing in that it contends the totality of the spiritual realm and operates outside of the belief that suffering is the sole result of physical or psychological causes (Taylor, 1997). As such, it contains elements of what might be called magic since there might appear to be an ineffable force at work (Bouse, 2017). A physician performs protocols to heal ills of the physical body, but spiritual healing claims to facilitate the opening of the pathway between the patient and the divine, thus allowing the patient to heal him or herself (Achterberg, 2002; Harrington, 2008; Taylor, 1997). The nature of spiritual healing is anomalous to the biomedical model that dominates contemporary Western culture, whereas medically verified instances of successful spiritual healing through shamanism, Christian Science, so-called miracles, psi, or other spiritual applications are perceived as extraordinary singularities (Krippner & Achterberg, 2014).

Healings performed by shamans demonstrate the need for the presence of belief in the efficacy of spiritual healing and the existence of a resonant worldview between the healer and the patient for effective healing to occur (Achterberg, 2002; Harrington, 2008; Krippner & Achterberg, 2014; Lipton, 2008; Taylor, 1997). Whether it be spiritual healing, herbal healing, or guided imagery (Wood & Patricolo, 2013), the common denominator in anomalous healing events is the commonality of belief (Craffert, 2012; Hutch, 2013; Schlitz, 2014). Cross-culturally, alternative healing protocols (including spiritual healing) are dependent on the belief in the efficacy of the actions of the healer by the patient (Ting, 2012).

The concept that spirituality and the intercession of the divine to effect healing of the mind and physical body does not solely belong to the domain of archaic or indigenous peoples. Judeo-Christian religions include instances of healing by faith (Carter, 2010; Kim, 2010; Kornu, 2014; Sharabi & Guzman-Carmeli, 2013; Tyler, 2013). Spiritual healings frequently require rituals in which the sacred is isolated and contained for the purpose of separating it from the mundane as evidenced in some

Native American ceremonies (Horowitz, 2012; Hultkrantz, 1992; Roseman, 2015). With increasing frequency, the importance of the spiritual history of the patient is also being recognized as relevant to his or her healing. According to Hart (2013) and Kirner (2014), 20% of clinical therapists report asking their patients to delve into their religious/spiritual orientations as part of psychotherapy.

In Closing

Neo-shamanic practice could have value as an adjunct to contemporary mental health practices because of its use in treating the spiritual aspect of mental distress and aiding contemporary therapists in standard clinical and humanistic practices to integrate the patient's spiritual aspect with their mental and physical states. In order to accomplish this effectively, Neo-shamanic practitioners and their potential therapeutic partners might benefit by going through an educational protocol to standardize some practices, establish a strong Code of Ethics, and assist individual practitioners in the deconstruction and resolution of issues present in their own psychologies in order to avoid spiritual bypassing and other pitfalls that could pose risks to their own psychological well-being and continued mental health.

The Big Question: What If?

The use of Neo-shamanic journey technique in a controlled laboratory setting for the purpose of consciousness research has the potential to provide a valid phenomenological database. From the standpoint of social science, using Neo-shamanic techniques in order to construct a phenomenological database holds considerable promise for the reason that the data gathered is generated simultaneously to the phenomenological experience rather than being recounted as an anecdote after the fact. For this reason, it holds promise as a research tool because of its potential to:

1. Create a baseline of phenomena that occur during shamanic journeys;
2. Offer insight into the lifeworlds of participants and perhaps expand the parameters of "normal" within the context of the current psychological paradigm; and
3. Isolate those phenomena that stand out as anomalous and independent of any potential cultural or internal genesis.

It is the last group of phenomena that offer researchers the richest foundation of further inquiry. For if these phenomena are not the products of personal history, culture, ethnic, or spiritual derivation, where did they come from?

Thomas Kuhn's *The Structure of Scientific Revolutions* (1996) presented a model of scientific change. The essence of Kuhn's theory is that when a dominant belief system fails to explain a pressing question or set of questions based on observed phenomena (a/k/a anomalies), the explanations derived from the study of the anomalies constitute a new dominant belief system or paradigm (Kuhn, 1996). A good example of this would be the observed anomaly of the orbit of Mars in the geocentric Ptolemaic model. The anomaly of Mars' periodic retrograde motion intrigued Copernicus, who subsequently discovered the heliocentric model of the solar system in his quest to discover the reason for Mars' periodic erratic behavior. The Copernican model constituted what Kuhn referred to as a scientific revolution because it changed the dominant astronomical paradigm (DeWitt, 2010). It also landed Copernicus in the loving arms of the Inquisition.

The entire premise of psychology from the time of Freud is that everything that we feel and perceive comes from within us. Under this paradigm, our dreams, fantasies, and illusions are the products of our minds processing traumas, repressed memories, and unfulfilled desires. Reality is restricted by the material world and what can be ascertained through the physical senses. Since psychology is the product of a culture that is based on rationalism, materialism, and positivistic science, it is no surprise that it developed in accordance with the caveats of mainstream culture. Jung's desire to incorporate the so-called paranormal into part of psychology's scientific covenant was a source of debate and eventual antagonism with his mentor Freud (Bair, 2003; McGuire, 1979). Over a century ago, Freud's conviction that psychology needed to conform to the scientific and medical models of the day in order to acquire legitimacy proved to dictate the course of development of the fledgling discipline. It has operated from within that paradigm ever since. It holds that anomalous phenomena are the products of our individual minds. Perception of anomalous visual and aural phenomena that are not included within our paradigmatic parameters of material sensory cognition is negated at best and pathologized at worst.

And yet these phenomena continue to be perceived and frequently reported formally or privately. They are the stuff of dreams, of journeys, of drug-induced experiences, of vision quests, and of food and sensory deprivation (Krippner & Friedman, 2010; Luke, 2017) in which the normal waking sensory apparatus is compromised to greater or lesser degree. They are alluded to in the Bible and other sacred works of faith and by people close to death or by those who have had near-death experiences. They are reported by people who have had close encounters with so-called aliens (Kripal, 2010; Streiber & Kripal, 2016). They are the worldwide subject of mythologies, legends, folktales, and songs. The common denominators underlying these reports are that:

- The perceivers believed the phenomena and experiences to be real.
- The anomalous events were frequently accompanied by some level of altered consciousness by the perceiver which allowed them to perceive the phenomena (Rock & Krippner, 2007).
- The perceivers sensed the phenomena to be something existing externally and separate from them.
- They are repetitive through time, geography, and cross-culturally (Winkelman, 2010).

From the mass phenomena of the Marian apparitions to the more personal experiences of people in journey, trance, or dream states, they frequently come with messages or have specific meaning to those who perceive them. They have been reported and preserved in the folktales, art, and literature of countless societies from the Paleolithic to the present day. Anomalous phenomena and experiences have been a part of human life for as long as we have been here. They have been accepted as honored and sacred life experiences in countless cultures worldwide (Winkelman, 2010). What is curious is that current Western society has marginalized and negated these occurrences and those who have experienced them.

Despite the dominant paradigm, anthropologists and psychologists have continued to find anomalous experiences both fascinating and significant. They have been the subject of valuable research by respected contemporary researchers. Among some of the most prominent are astrophysicist Jacques Vallee, physicist Dean Radin, anthropologist Michael Winkelman, religionist Jeffrey Kripal, and psychologists Stanley Krippner, Etzel Cardena, and Adam Rock. Their findings have positively reinforced the concept that anomalous experiences occur to people of all ages, cultures, and walks of life and have sown the seeds of what may potentially be the beginning of a paradigm shift which would incorporate the idea that anomalous experiences are real and perhaps may not be internally generated projections of unresolved personal traumas and repressed desires. Rather, they may be witnessed interceptions with the mundane material world and phenomena that originate and reside outside of the boundaries of our sensory cognitive capacities to perceive them.

The shamans of ancient and indigenous cultures used the journey technique to personally interface with the world outside of sensory cognition in order to bring healing, wisdom, and insight to the members of the tribe or community. With the help of the spirits, they eased souls through the transitions of birth, maturation, and death. Shamanism is a global practice and belief system that has transcended time, geography, and culture. Perhaps it is possible that by using their technologies as revitalized and currently practiced by Neo-shamans in the name of therapy, personal discovery, and research, psychologists might just help to provide a window into the answers of some of humanity's most enduring existential questions.

References

Achterberg, J. (2002). *Imagery in healing: Shamanism and modern medicine.* Boulder, CO: Shambhala.

Bair, D. (2003). *Jung: A biography.* New York, NY: Back Bay Books.

Bouse, K. (2017). *Neo-shamanism as a developmental, spiritual matrix for contemporary magical discovery and practice* (Doctoral dissertation). Available from ProQuest Dissertations and Theses database (No. 10742675).

Carter, W. (2010). Jesus's healing stories: Imperial critiques and eschatological anticipations in Matthew's Gospel. *Currents in Theology and Mission, 37*(6), 488–496.

Craffert, P. (2012). The placebo phenomenon and well-being: Notes on the healing process as an evolutionary adaptive trait. *Religion & Theology, 19,* 181–203.

DeWitt, R. (2010). *Worldview: An introduction to the history and philosophy of science* (2nd ed.). Chichester, UK: Wiley-Blackwell.

Harner, S. (2005). Presence in existential-humanistic psychotherapy and in the shamanic journey. *International Institute for Humanistic Studies.* http://www.human-studies.com.

Harrington, A. (2008). *The cure within: A history of mind-body medicine.* New York, NY: W. W. Norton.

Hart, J. (2013). Tools for exploring patients' spirituality. *Alternative and Complementary Therapies, 19*(4), 202–204.

Horowitz, S. (2012). American Indian health: Integrating traditional native healing practices with Western medicine. *Alternative and Contemporary Therapies, 18*(1), 24–30.

Hultkrantz, A. (1992). *Shamanic healing and ritual drama: Health and medicine in native North American religious traditions.* New York, NY: Crossroad.

Hutch, R. (2013). Health and healing: Spiritual, pharmaceutical, and mechanical medicine. *Journal of Religion and Health, 52,* 955–965.

Kim, S. (2010). The significance of Jesus's healing the blind man in John 9. *Bibliotheca Sacra, 167,* 307–318.

Kirner, K. (2014). Healing community: Pagan cultural models and experiences in seeking well-being. *The Pomegranate, 16*(1), 80–108.

Kornu, K. (2014). The beauty of healing: Covenant, eschatology, and Jonathan Edwards' theological aesthetics toward a theology of medicine. *Christian Bioethics, 20*(1), 43–58.

Kripal, J. (2010). *Authors of the impossible: The paranormal and the sacred.* Chicago, IL: University of Chicago Press.

Krippner, S., & Achterberg, J. (2014). Anomalous healing experiences. In E. Cardena, S. Lynn, & S. Krippner (Eds.), *Varieties of anomalous experiences: Examining the scientific evidence* (2nd ed., pp. 273–302). Washington, DC: American Psychological Association.

Krippner, S., & Friedman, H. (Eds.). (2010). *Mysterious minds: The neurobiology of psychics, mediums and other extraordinary people.* Santa Barbara, CA: Praeger.

Kuhn, T. (1996). *The structure of scientific revolutions* (3rd ed.). Chicago, IL: University of Chicago Press.

Lipton, B. (2008). *The biology of belief: Unleashing the power of consciousness, matter & miracles.* New York, NY: Hay House.

Luke, D. (2017). *Otherworlds: Psychedelics and exceptional human experiences.* London, UK: Muswell Hill Press.

Mackinnon, C. (2012). *Shamanism and spirituality in therapeutic practice.* London, UK: Singing Dragon.

McClenon, J. (1997). Shamanic healing, human evolution and the origin of religion. *Journal for the Scientific Study of Religion, 36*(3), 345–354.

McGuire, W. (Ed.). (1979). *The Freud and Jung letters.* Princeton, NJ: Princeton University Press.

Rock, A., & Krippner, S. (2007). Shamanism and the confusion of consciousness with phenomenological content. *North American Journal of Psychology, 9*(3), 485–500.

Roseman, J. (2015). Creating sacred space: Spirituality in the medical encounter—Part 1. *Alternative and Contemporary Therapies, 22*(6), 247–254.

Schlitz, M. (2014). Transpersonal healing: Assessing the evidence form laboratory and clinical trials. *International Journal of Transpersonal Studies, 33*(1), 97–101.

Sharabi, A., & Guzman-Carmeli, S. (2013). The Teshuva bargain: Ritual healing performances at Rabbi Amnon Yitzchak's rallies. *The Journal of Ritual Studies, 27*(2), 97–110.

Streiber, W., & Kripal, J. (2016). *The supernatural: A new vision of the unexplained*. New York, NY: Jeremy P. Tarcher/Penguin.

Taylor, E. (1997). *A psychology of spiritual healing*. West Chester, PA: Chrysalis.

Ting, R. (2012). The worldviews of healing traditions in the East and West: Implications for psychology of religion. *Pastoral Psychology, 61*, 759–782.

Tyler, K. (2013). Principles of Jesus's healing ministry. *Journal of Applied Christian Leadership, 7*(2), 8–20.

Winkelman, M. (2010). *Shamanism: A biopsychosocial paradigm of consciousness and healing* (2nd ed.). Santa Barbara, CA: Praeger.

Wood, D., & Patricolo, G. (2013). Using guided imagery in a hospital setting. *Alternative and Complementary Therapies, 19*(6), 301–305.

Bibliography

Achterberg, J. (2002). *Imagery in healing: Shamanism and modern medicine*. Boulder, CO: Shambhala.

Aldred, L. (2000). Plastic shamans and Astroturf sun dances: New age commercialization of Native American spirituality. *American Indian Quarterly, 24*(3), 329–352.

Amarasingarn, A. (2009). New age spirituality, quantum mysticism and self-psychology: Changing ourselves from the inside out. *Mental Health, Religion & Culture, 12*(3), 277–287.

American Psychiatric Association. (2013). *Diagnostic and statistical manual of mental disorders, 5th edition: DSM-5*. Alexandria, VA: American Psychiatric Association.

Armstrong, T. (2010). *The power of neurodiversity: Unleashing the advantage of your differently wired brain*. Cambridge, MA: Da Capo Press.

Avalos, H. (2014). Nebuchadnezzar's affliction: New Mesopotamian parallels for Daniel 4. *Journal of Biblical Literature, 133*(3), 497–507.

Bair, D. (2003). *Jung: A biography*. New York, NY: Back Bay Books.

Bartolini, N., Chris, R., MacKian, S., & Pile, S. (2013). Psychics, crystals, candels, and cauldrons: Alternative spiritualities and the question of their esoteric economics. *Social & Cultural Geography, 14*(4), 367–388.

Becker, E. (1973). *The denial of death*. New York, NY: Free Press Paperback.

Berger, H. (2005). Witchcraft and neo-paganism. In H. Berger (Ed.), *Witchcraft and magic: Contemporary North America* (pp. 28–54). Philadelphia, PA: University of Pennsylvania Press.

Berger, P., & Luckmann, T. (1996). *The social construction of reality: A treatise on the sociology of knowledge*. New York, NY: Anchor.

K. J. Bouse, *Neo-shamanism and Mental Health*,
https://doi.org/10.1007/978-3-030-31911-3

Bird, E. (2005). Going native or going naïve? Shamanism and the neo-noble savage. *Great Plains Quarterly, 25*(1), 60.

Bogzaran, F., & Deslauriers, D. (2012). *Integral dreaming: A holistic approach to dreams.* Albany, NY: SUNY Press.

Bouse, K. (2017). *Neo-shamanism as a developmental, spiritual matrix for contemporary magical discovery and practice* (Doctoral dissertation). Available from ProQuest Dissertations and Theses database (No. 10742675).

Cambray, J., & Carter, L. (Eds.). (2004). *Analytical psychology: Contemporary perspectives in Jungian analysis.* New York, NY: Routledge.

Campbell, J. (1959). *Primitive mythology: The masks of God* (Vol. 1). New York, NY: Penguin.

Campbell, J. (1973). *The hero with a thousand faces.* Princeton, NJ: Princeton University Press.

Cardena, E. (2011). Altered consciousness in emotion and psychopathology. In E. Cardena & M. Winkelman (Eds.), *Altering consciousness: Multidisciplinary perspectives, vol. 2: Biological and psychological perspectives* (pp. 279–300). Santa Barbara, CA: Praeger.

Cardena, E., & Krippner, S. (2010). The cultural context of hypnosis. In S. Lynn, J. Rhue, & J. Kirsch (Eds.), *Handbook of clinical hypnosis* (pp. 743–772). Washington, DC: American Psychological Association.

Cardena, E., Lynn, S., & Krippner, S. (2014). Introduction: Anomalous experiences in perspective. In E. Cardena, S. Lynn, & S. Krippner (Eds.), *Varieties of anomalous experience: Examining the scientific evidence* (2nd ed., pp. 3–20). Washington, DC: American Psychological Association.

Carkhuff, R. (2009). *The art of helping* (9th ed.). Amherst, MA: Possibilities Publishing Inc.

Carter, W. (2010). Jesus's healing stories: Imperial critiques and eschatological anticipations in Matthew's Gospel. *Currents in Theology and Mission, 37*(6), 488–496.

Cartwright, R. (2010). *The twenty-four hour mind: The role of sleep and dreaming in our emotional lives.* New York, NY: Oxford University Press.

Cheyne, J. (1982). Sleep paralysis and the structure of waking nightmare hallucinations. *Dreaming, 13*(3), 163–179.

Clarke, P., Giordano, A., Cashwell, C., & Lewis, T. (2013). The straight path to healing: Using motivational interviewing to address spiritual bypass. *Journal of Counseling and Development, 91,* 87–94.

Claridge, G. (2001). Spiritual experience: Healthy psychoticism? In I. Clarke (Ed.), *Psychosis and spirituality: Exploring the New Frontier* (pp. 90–106). Philadelphia, PA: Whurr Publishers.

Clifton, C. (2003). Smokey and the sacred: Nature, religion, civil religion and American Paganism. *Ecotheology, 8*(1), 50–60.

Colman, A. (Ed.). (2009). *Oxford dictionary of psychology* (3rd ed.). New York, NY: Oxford University Press.

Craffert, P. (2012). The placebo phenomenon and well-being: Notes on the healing process as an evolutionary adaptive trait. *Religion & Theology, 19,* 181–203.

Crockford, S. (2011). Entering the crack between the worlds: Symbolism in Western shamanism. *The Pomegranate, 13*(2), 184–204.

Csikszentmihalyi, M. (1996). *Creativity: The psychology of discovery and invention.* New York, NY: Harper Perennial.

DeConick, A. (2016). *The Gnostic new age: How a countercultural spirituality revolutionized religion from antiquity to today.* New York, NY: Columbia University Press.

DeWitt, R. (2010). *Worldview: An introduction to the history and philosophy of science* (2nd ed.). Chichester, UK: Wiley-Blackwell.

DuBois, T. (2011). Trends in contemporary research on shamanism. *Numen, 58,* 100–128.

Eliade, M. (1964). *Shamanism: Archaic techniques of ecstasy.* Princeton, NJ: Princeton University Press.

Erikson, E. (1980). *Identity and the life cycle.* New York, NY: W. W. Norton.

Eskenazi, E. (2010). *The roots of new age spirituality in United States social history* (Doctoral dissertation). Available from ProQuest Dissertations and Theses Global (UMI No. 88897031).

Feinstein, D., & Krippner, S. (2006). *The mythic path* (3rd ed.). Ashland, OR: Innersource.

Fiere, S., & Kirbis, A. (2009a). New age is not inimical to religion and traditionalism. *Journal for the Scientific Study of Religion, 48*(1), 161–169.

Fiere, S., & Kirbis, A. (2009b). New age, religiosity, and traditionalism: A cross-cultural comparison. *Journal for the Scientific Study of Religion, 48*(1), 179–184.

Fox, J., Cashwell, C., & Picciotto, G. (2017). The opiate of the masses: Measuring spiritual bypass and its relationship to spirituality, religion, mindfulness, psychological distress and personality. *Spirituality in Clinical Practice, 4*(4), 274–287.

Fuller, R. (2001). *Spiritual but not religious: Understanding unchurched America.* New York, NY: Oxford University Press.

Furlong, D. (2014). *Healing your ancestral patterns: How to access the past to heal the present.* Malvern, Worcestershire, UK: Atlanta Books.

Gadamer, H.-G. (1975). *Truth and method.* New York, NY: Bloomsbury.

Garrod, A., Smulyom, C., Powers, S., & Kilkenny, R. (2008). *Adolescent portraits: Identity, relationships, and challenges.* New York, NY: Hill Higher Education.

Gawryluk, J., D'Arcy, R., Connolly, J., & Weaver, D. (2010). Improving the clinical assessment of consciousness with advances in electrophysiological and neuroimaging techniques. *BMC Neurology, 10,* 1–7.

Geels, A. (2011). Altered consciousness in religion. In E. Cardena & M. Winkelman (Eds.), *Altering consciousness: Multidisciplinary perspectives, vol. 1: History, culture and the humanities* (pp. 255–276). Santa Barbara, CA: Praeger.

Geertz, C. (1973). *The interpretation of cultures*. New York, NY: Basic.

Goulding, A. (2005). Healthy schizotypy in a population of paranormal believers and experiments. *Personality and Individual Differences, 38*(5), 1069–1083.

Granqvist, P., Hagekull, B., & Ivarsson, T. (2012). Disorganized attachment promotes mystical experiences via a propensity for alterations in consciousness (absorption). *The International Journal for the Psychology of Religion, 22*(3), 180–197.

Grof, S. (2006). *When the impossible happens: Adventures in non-ordinary realities*. Boulder, CO: Sounds True.

Harner, M. (1982). *The way of the shaman*. New York, NY: Bantam.

Harner, M. (2005). The history and work of the Foundation for Shamanic Studies. *Shamanism (25th Anniversary Issue), 18*(1–2). Available at http://www.shamanism.org/articles/article18.html.

Harner, M. (2014). *Cave and cosmos*. Berkeley, CA: North Atlantic.

Harner, S. (2005). Presence in existential-humanistic psychotherapy and in the shamanic journey. *International Institute for Humanistic Studies*. http://www.human-studies.com.

Harrelson, W. (Ed.). (2003). *The new interpreter's study Bible: New revised standard version with the Apocrypha*. Nashville, TN: Abingdon Press.

Harrington, A. (2008). *The cure within: A history of mind-body medicine*. New York, NY: W. W. Norton.

Harris, M. (1979). *Cultural materialism: The struggle for a science of culture*. New York, NY: Vintage.

Harrow, J. (2002). *Spiritual mentoring: A pagan guide*. Toronto, ON, Canada: ECW.

Hart, J. (2013). Tools for exploring patients' spirituality. *Alternative and Complementary Therapies, 19*(4), 202–204.

Herbert, R. (2011). Reconsidering music and trance: Cross-cultural differences and cross-disciplinary perspectives. *Ethnomusicology Forum, 20*(2), 201–227.

Hinton, D., Hufford, D., & Kirmayer, L. (2005). Culture and sleep paralysis. *Transcultural Psychiatry, 42*(1), 5–10.

Hood, R. (2013). Theory and methods in the psychological study of mysticism. *International Journal for the Psychology of Religion, 23*(4), 294–306.

Hood, R., Hill, P., & Spilka, B. (2009). *The psychology of religion: An empirical approach* (4th ed.). New York, NY: Guilford.

Horowitz, S. (2012). American Indian health: Integrating traditional native healing practices with Western medicine. *Alternative and Contemporary Therapies, 18*(1), 24–30.

House, R. (2001). Psychopathology, psychosis and the kundalini: Postmodern perspectives on unusual subjective experience. In I. Clarke (Ed.), *Psychosis and spirituality: Exploring the New Frontier* (pp. 107–125). Philadelphia, PA: Whurr Publishers.

Hufford, D. (1989). *The terror that comes in the night: An experienced centered study of supernatural assault traditions.* Philadelphia, PA: University of Philadelphia Press.

Hufford, D. (2005). Sleep paralysis and spiritual experience. *Transcultural Psychiatry, 42*(1), 46–77.

Hultkrantz, A. (1992). *Shamanic healing and ritual drama: Health and medicine in native North American religious traditions.* New York, NY: Crossroad.

Hunt, H. (2010). Consciousness and society: Societal aspects and implications of transpersonal psychology. *International Journal of Transpersonal Studies, 29*(1), 20–30.

Hutch, R. (2013). Health and healing: Spiritual, pharmaceutical, and mechanical medicine. *Journal of Religion & Health, 52,* 955–965.

Hutton, R. (2010). Writing the history of witchcraft: A personal view. *The Pomegranate, 12*(2), 239–262.

Hutton, R. (2011). Revisionism and counter revisionism in Pagan history. *The Pomegranate, 13*(2), 255–256.

Irwin, H. (1990). Fantasy proneness and paranormal beliefs. *Psychological Reports, 66*(2), 655–658.

Irwin, H. (2009). *The psychology of paranormal belief: A researcher's handbook.* Hatfield, Hertfordshire, UK: University of Hertfordshire Press.

Jacobi, J. (1973). *The psychology of C. G. Jung.* New Haven, CT: Yale University Press.

James, W. (1902). *The varieties of religious experience.* New York, NY: Barnes & Noble.

Jones, S., & Krippner, S. (2012). *The voice of Rolling Thunder: A medicine man's wisdom for walking the red road.* Rochester, VT: Bear & Company.

Jonsson, K., Grim, K., & Kjellgren, A. (2014). Do highly sensitive persons experience more nonordinary states of consciousness during sensory isolation? *Social Behavior and Personality: An International Journal, 42,* 1495–1506. https://doi.org/10.2224/sbp.2014.42.9.1495.

Jourdain, R. (2002). *Music, the brain, and ecstasy: How music captures our imagination.* New York, NY: Quill/Harper Collins.

Jung, C. (1961). *Memories, dreams, reflections.* New York, NY: Vintage.

Jung, C. (1964). *Man and his symbols.* New York, NY: Doubleday.

Jung, C. (1966). *Two essays in analytical psychology.* Princeton, NJ: Princeton University Press.

Jung, C. (1967). *Alchemical studies.* Princeton, NJ: Princeton University Press.

Jung, C. (1968). *Psychology and alchemy.* Princeton, NJ: Princeton University Press.

Jung, C. (1974). *Dreams*. Princeton, NJ: Princeton University Press.

Jung, C. (2009). *The red book: Liber novus*. New York, NY: W. W. Norton.

Kim, S. (2010). The significance of Jesus's healing the blind man in John 9. *Bibliotheca Sacra, 167,* 307–318.

Kirner, K. (2014). Healing community: Pagan cultural models and experiences in seeking well-being. *The Pomegranate, 16*(1), 80–108.

Kjellgren, A., & Erickson, K. (2013). Methoxetamine (MXE)–A phenomenological study of experiences induced by a "legal high" from the internet. *Journal of Psychoactive Drugs, 45*(3), 276–286. https://doi.org/10.1080/02791072.2013.803647.

Kokoszka, A., & Wallace, B. (2011). Sleep, dreams, and other biological cycles in altered states of consciousness. In E. Cardena & M. Winkelman (Eds.), *Altering consciousness: Multidisciplinary perspectives, vol. 2: Biological and psychological perspectives* (pp. 3–20). Santa Barbara, CA: Praeger.

Kornu, K. (2014). The beauty of healing: Covenant, eschatology, and Jonathan Edwards' theological aesthetics toward a theology of medicine. *Christian Bioethics, 20*(1), 43–58.

Kremer, J. (2004). (Post) modern brain—shaman's brain: Evolutionary perspectives on shamanic processes and potentials. In D. Eigner (Ed.), *Consciousness: Cultural and therapeutic perspectives* (pp. 47–75). Frankfurt am Main, DE: Peter Lang International.

Kremer, J., & Jackson-Paton, R. (2014). *Ethno-autobiography*. Sebastopol, CA: ReVision.

Kripal, J. (2010). *Authors of the impossible: The paranormal and the sacred*. Chicago, IL: University of Chicago Press.

Krippner, S. (2000). The epistemologies and technologies of shamanic states of consciousness. *Journal of Consciousness Studies, 7,* 93–118.

Krippner, S., & Achterberg, J. (2014). Anomalous healing experiences. In E. Cardena, S. Lynn, & S. Krippner (Eds.), *Varieties of anomalous experiences: Examining the scientific evidence* (2nd ed., pp. 273–302). Washington, DC: American Psychological Association.

Krippner, S., & Friedman, H. (Eds.). (2010). *Mysterious minds: The neurobiology of psychics, mediums and other extraordinary people*. Santa Barbara, CA: Praeger.

Krishna, G. (1971). *Kundalini: The evolutionary energy in man*. Boston, MA: Shambhala Publications.

Kuhn, T. (1996). *The structure of scientific revolutions* (3rd ed.). Chicago, IL: University of Chicago Press.

Langdon, E., & Santana De Rose, I. (2012). (Neo) shamanic dialogues. *Nova Religio, 15*(4), 36–59.

Leahey, T. (2013). *A history of psychology: From antiquity to modernity*. Boston, MA: Pearson.

Leuchter, M. (2015). Jehoiakim and the scribes: A note on Jer 36, 23. *Zeitschrift fur die alttestamenthliche Wissenschaft, 127*(2), 320–325.

Linton, M. (2015). Altered states of consciousness and creative expression. *International Journal of Transpersonal Studies, 34*(1–2), 98–102.

Lipton, B. (2008). *The biology of belief: Unleashing the power of consciousness, matter & miracles.* New York, NY: Hay House.

Llamazares, A. (2015). The wounded west: The healing potential of shamanism in the contemporary world. *ReVision, 23*(2&3), 6–23.

Luhrmann, T. (2012). Touching the divine: Recent research on neo-paganism and neo-shamanism. *Reviews in Anthropology, 41,* 136–150.

Luke, D. (2012). Psychoactive substances and paranormal phenomena: A comprehensive review. *International Journal of Transpersonal Studies, 31*(1), 97–156.

Luke, D. (2017). *Otherworlds: Psychedelics and exceptional human experiences.* London, UK: Muswell Hill Press.

Lukoff, D. (2011). Visionary spirituality and mental disorders. In E. Cardena & M. Winkelman (Eds.), *Altering consciousness: Multidisciplinary perspectives, vol. 2: Biological and psychological perspectives* (pp. 301–326). Santa Barbara, CA: Praeger.

Lynn, S., & Rhue, J. (1986). The fantasy-prone person: Hypnosis, imagination, and creativity. *Journal of Personality and Social Psychology, 51*(2), 404–408.

MacDonald, D. (2012). Spiritual identity: Individual perspectives. In S. Schwartz, K. Luyckx, & V. Vignoles (Eds.), *Handbook of identity theory and research* (Vol. 2, pp. 531–562). New York, NY: Springer.

Magliocco, S. (2004). *Witching culture: Folklore and neo-paganism in America.* Philadelphia, PA: University of Pennsylvania Press.

Malan, G. (2016). Mythology, weltanschauung, symbolic universe, and states of consciousness. *Hervormde Teologiese Studies, 72*(1), 1–8.

Masters, A. (2010). *Spiritual bypassing: When spirituality disconnects us from what really matters.* Berkeley, CA: North Atlantic.

Mayer, G. (2013). Spirituality and extraordinary experiences: Methodological remarks and some empirical findings. *Journal of Empirical Theology, 26*(2), 188–206.

McAdams, D. (2012). Narrative identity. In S. Schwartz, K. Luyckx, & V. Vignoles (Eds.), *Handbook of identity theory and research* (Vol. 1, pp. 99–115). New York, NY: Springer.

McClenon, J. (1997). Shamanic healing, human evolution and the origin of religion. *Journal for the Scientific Study of Religion, 36*(3), 345–354.

McClenon, J. (2011). A community survey of psychological symptoms: Evaluating evolutionary theories regarding shamanism and schizophrenia. *Mental Health, Religion & Culture, 15*(8), 799–816.

McCrae, M. (2019). *Medicinal herbs used in the civil war found blast drug resistant bacteria in the lab.* https://sciencealert.com.

McGuire, W. (Ed.). (1979). *The Freud and Jung letters*. Princeton, NJ: Princeton University Press.

McKinnon, C. (2012). *Shamanism and spirituality in therapeutic practice*. London, UK: Singing Dragon.

McNamara, P. (2004). *An evolutionary psychology of sleep and dreams*. Westport, CT: Praeger.

Mears, D. (2000). Who buys new age materials? Exploring sociodemographic, religious network, and contextual correlates of new age consumption. *Sociology of Religion, 61*(3), 289–313.

Mellick, J. (2019). Piercing the mundane: The role of creative expression in transpersonal psychology. *The Journal of Transpersonal Psychology, 50*, 144–159.

Merckelbach, H., Horselenberg, R., & Muris, P. (2001). The creative experiences questionnaire (CEQ): A brief self-report measure of fantasy proneness. *Personality and Individual Differences, 31*, 987–995.

Mitchell, S., Price, N., Hutton, R., Purkiss, D., Patton, K., Raudvere, C., … Sepulveda, V. (2013). Wicca and neo-paganism: A primer for counselors. *Journal of Professional Counseling: Practice, Theory and Research, 40*(1), 38–48.

Mohr, C., & Claridge, G. (2015). Schizotypy—Do not worry, it is not all worrisome. *Schizophrenia Bulletin, 4*(2), S436–S443.

Morgaine, R. (2013). The alchemy of life: Magic, anthropology and human nature in Pagan theology. *Australian Journal of Anthropology, 24*(3), 290–309.

Moustakas, C. (1994a). *Existential psychotherapy and the interpretation of dreams*. Northvale, NJ: Jason Aronson.

Moustakas, C. (1994b). *Phenomenological research methods*. Thousand Oaks, CA: Sage.

Nelson, J. (2009). *Psychology, religion, and spirituality*. New York, NY: Springer.

Orgel, S., & Braunmuller, A. (Eds.). (2002). *William Shakespeare: The complete works*. New York, NY: Penguin Books.

Pekala, R. J. (1991). *Quantifying consciousness: Emotions, personality, and psychotherapy*. Boston, MA: Springer.

Polimeni, J. (2012). *Shamans among us: Schizophrenia, shamanism and the evolutionary origins of religion*. Sao Paulo, Brazil: Evo.

Revonsuo, A. (2009a). Inner presence: Consciousness as a biological phenomenon. Cambridge, MA: MIT Press.

Revonsuo, A. (2009b). What is an altered state of consciousness? *Philosophical Psychology, 22*(2), 187.

Richards, R. (2001). Creativity and the schizophrenic spectrum: More and more interesting. *Creativity Research Journal, 13*(1), 111–132.

Richards, R. (2009). Everyday creativity and psychopathology. *Psychological Inquiry, 4*(3), 212–217.

Richards, R. (2018). *Everyday creativity and the healthy mind: Dynamic new paths for self and society*. London, UK: Palgrave Macmillan.

Richards, R., & Kinney, D. (1990). Mood swings and creativity. *Creativity Research Journal, 3*(3), 202–217.

Ripinsky-Naxon, M. (1993). *The nature of shamanism*. Albany, NY: SUNY Press.

Rock, A. (2006). Phenomenological analysis of experimentally induced visual mental imagery associated with shamanic journeying to the lower world. *International Journal of Transpersonal Psychology, 25*, 45–55.

Rock, A., & Baynes, P. (2005). Shamanic journeying imagery, constructivism, and the affect of bridge technique. *Anthropology of Consciousness, 16*(2), 50–71.

Rock, A., & Baynes, P. (2007). What are the origins of shamanic journeying imagery? The modification of hypnoanalytic technique to address and enduring methodological problem. *The Humanistic Psychologist, 35*(4), 349–361.

Rock, A., & Casey, P. (2005). Experimental study of ostensibly shamanic journeying imagery in naïve participants I: Antecedents. *Anthropology of Consciousness, 16*(2), 72–92.

Rock, A., Casey, P., & Baynes, P. (2006). Experimental study of ostensibly shamanic journey imagery in naive participants II: Phenomenological mapping and modified effect bridge. *Anthropology of Consciousness, 17*(1), 65–83.

Rock, A., & Krippner, S. (2007a). Does the concept of "altered states of consciousness" rest on a mistake? *International Journal of Transpersonal Studies, 26*, 303–340.

Rock, A., & Krippner, S. (2007b). Shamanism and the confusion of consciousness with phenomenological content. *North American Journal of Psychology, 9*(3), 485–500.

Rock, A., & Krippner, S. (2008a). Is a realistic interpretation of shamanic nonphysical worlds logically incoherent? *Transpersonal Psychology Review, 12*(2), 23–31.

Rock, A., & Krippner, S. (2008b). Proposed criteria for the necessary conditions for shamanic journeying inquiry. *Journal of Scientific Exploration, 22*(2), 215–226.

Rock, A., & Krippner, S. (2008c). Some rudimentary problems pertaining to the construction of an ontology and epistemology of shamanic journeying imagery. *International Journal of Transpersonal Psychology, 27*, 12–19.

Rock, A., & Krippner, S. (2011). *Demystifying shamans and their world: An interdisciplinary study*. Charlottesville, VA: Imprint Academic.

Rock, A., Abbott, G., Childargushi, H., & Kiehne, M. (2008). The effects of shamanic like stimulus conditions and the cognitive-perceptual factor of schizotypy on phenomenology. *North American Journal of Psychology, 10*(1), 79–98.

Roseman, J. (2015). Creating sacred space: Spirituality in the medical encounter—Part 1. *Alternative and Contemporary Therapies, 22*(6), 247–254.

Sacks, O. (2007). *Musicophilia: Tales of music and the brain*. New York, NY: Vintage Books.

Sala, L. (2014). *Ritual: A magical perspective*. New Delhi, IN: Nirala.

Santrock, J. (2009). *Life-span development.* New York, NY: McGraw-Hill Higher Education.

Sarasola, C. (2015). Reality, invisible world, and shamanism: An outlook from an indigenous worldview. *ReVision, 17*(2–3), 24–31.

Saunders, R. (2012). Pagan places: Towards a religiosity of neopaganism. *Progress in Human Geography, 37*(6), 786–810.

Schlitz, M. (2014). Transpersonal healing: Assessing the evidence form laboratory and clinical trials. *International Journal of Transpersonal Studies, 33*(1), 97–101.

Schwab, J. (2010). *Haunting legacies: Violent histories and transgenerational trauma.* New York, NY: Columbia University Press.

Segal, R. (1992). *The Gnostic Jung.* London, UK: Routledge.

Shamdasani, S. (2003). *Jung and the making of modern psychology: A dream of a science.* New York, NY: Cambridge University Press.

Sharabi, A., & Guzman-Carmeli, S. (2013). The Teshuva bargain: Ritual healing performances at Rabbi Amnon Yitzchak's rallies. *The Journal of Ritual Studies, 27*(2), 97–110.

Sidky, H. (2010). On the antiquity of shamanism and its role in human religiosity. *Method & Theory in the Study of Religion, 22*(1), 68–92.

Smith, C. (2007). *Jung and shamanism in dialogue.* New York, NY: Paulist.

St. John, G. (2011). Spiritual technologies and altering consciousness in contemporary counterculture. In E. Cardena & M. Winkelman (Eds.), *Altering consciousness: Multidisciplinary perspectives, vol. 1: History, culture and the humanities* (pp. 203–228). Santa Barbara, CA: Praeger.

Starhawk. (1979). *The spiral dance: A rebirth of the ancient religion of the great Goddess.* New York, NY: Harper & Row.

Stevens, A., & Price, J. (2006). *Evolutionary psychology: A new beginning* (2nd ed.). New York, NY: Routledge.

Streiber, W., & Kripal, J. (2016). *The supernatural: A new vision of the unexplained.* New York, NY: Jeremy P. Tarcher/Penguin.

Strmiska, M. (2004). Review of nine worlds of Seid-magic: Ecstasy and neo-shamanism in North European paganism by Jenny Blain. *Nova Religio, 7*(3), 99–101.

Sutton, P. (2010). Aboriginal spirituality in a new age. *Australian Journal of Anthropology, 21*(1), 71–89.

Taylor, E. (1997). *A psychology of spiritual healing.* West Chester, PA: Chrysalis.

Thomas, K. (1971). *Religion and the decline of magic.* New York, NY: Charles Scribner's Sons.

Thurber, J. (2016). *The secret life of Walter Mitty.* New York, NY: Penguin Press.

Ting, R. (2012). The worldviews of healing traditions in the East and West: Implications for psychology of religion. *Pastoral Psychology, 61,* 759–782.

Tucker, K. (2002). New age religion and the cult of the self. *Society*, January–February, 46–51.

Tyler, K. (2013). Principles of Jesus's healing ministry. *Journal of Applied Christian Leadership, 7*(2), 8–20.

Vaitl, D., Birbaumer, G., Gruzelier, J., Jamieson, G., & Kotchoubey, B. (2013). Psychobiology of altered states of consciousness. *Psychology of Consciousness: Theory, Research, and Practice, 1*(5), 2–47.

VandenBos, G. (Ed.). (2015). *APA dictionary of psychology* (2nd ed.). Washington, DC: American Psychological Association.

Versluis, A. (2014). *American gurus: From American transcendentalism to new age religion*. New York, NY: Oxford University Press.

Wallis, R. (2003). *Shamans/neo-shamans: Ecstasy, alternative archaeologies, and contemporary paganism*. London, UK: Routledge.

Walsh, R. (1992). *The spirit of shamanism*. Los Angeles, CA: Jeremy P. Tarcher Inc.

Welwood, J. (1979). Principles of inner work: Psychological and spiritual. *The Journal of Transpersonal Psychology, 16*(1), 63–73.

Weston, B. (2011). The new metaphysical: Spirituality and the American religious imagination. *Choice, 48*(5), 912–913.

Whisker, D. (2013). The possibility of shamanism: A genealogy of anthropological appropriations. *History and Anthropology, 24*(3), 344–362.

White, N. (2014). Devil's stones and midnight rites: Megaliths, folklore, and contemporary Pagan witchcraft. *Folklore, 125*, 60–79.

Williams, E., Francis, L., Billington, U., & Robbins, M. (2012). The psychological-type profile of practicing British druids compared with Anglican churchgoers. *Mental Health, Religion & Culture, 15*(10), 1065–1075.

Wilson, S., & Barber, T. (1982). The fantasy-prone personality: Implications for understanding imagery, hypnosis, and parapsychological phenomena. *PSI Research, 1*(3), 94–116.

Winkelman, M. (2004). Shamanism as the original neurotheology. *Zygon, 39*(1), 193–217.

Winkelman, M. (2009). Shamanism and the origins of spirituality and ritual healing. *Journal for the Study of Religion, Nature and Culture, 3*(4), 458–489.

Winkelman, M. (2010). *Shamanism: A biopsychosocial paradigm of consciousness and healing* (2nd ed.). Santa Barbara, CA: Praeger.

Winkelman, M. (2011a). A paradigm for understanding altered consciousness: The integrative role of consciousness. In E. Cardena & M. Winkelman (Eds.), *Altering consciousness: Multidisciplinary perspectives, vol. I: History, culture and the humanities* (pp. 23–44). Santa Barbara, CA: Praeger.

Winkelman, M. (2011b). Shamanism and the alteration of consciousness. In E. Cardena & M. Winkelman (Eds.), *Altering consciousness: Multidisciplinary perspectives, vol. 1: History, culture and the humanities* (pp. 159–180). Santa Barbara, CA: Praeger.

Winkelman, M. (2013a). Shamanic cosmology as an evolutionary neurocognitive epistemology. *International Journal of Transpersonal Studies, 23*(1), 79–99.

Winkelman, M. (2013b). Shamanism in cross-cultural perspective. *International Journal of Transpersonal Studies, 31*(2), 79–99.

Winkelman, M., & Baker, J. (2010). *Supernatural and natural: A biocultural approach to religion*. New York, NY: Routledge.

Wood, D., & Patricolo, G. (2013). Using guided imagery in a hospital setting. *Alternative and Complementary Therapies, 19*(6), 301–305.

Yin, R. (2009). *Case study research: Design and methods* (4th ed.). Los Angeles, CA: Sage.

York, M. (2002). *Pagan theology: Paganism as a world religion*. New York, NY: New York University Press.

York, M. (2005a). New age and magic. In H. Berger (Ed.), *Witchcraft and magic in contemporary North America* (pp. 8–28). Philadelphia, PA: University of Pennsylvania Press.

York, M. (2005b). Shamanism and magic. In H. Berger (Ed.), *Witchcraft and magic in contemporary North America* (pp. 81–101). Philadelphia, PA: University of Pennsylvania Press.

Zimdars-Schwartz, S. (1991). *Encountering Mary*. New York, NY: Avon.

Index

K. J. Bouse, *Neo-shamanism and Mental Health*,
https://doi.org/10.1007/978-3-030-31911-3